Core
Clinical
Cases in

Obstetrics and Gynaecology

Third edition

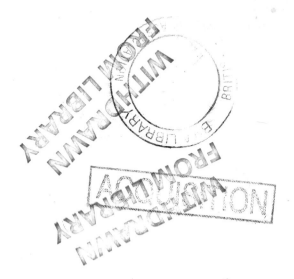

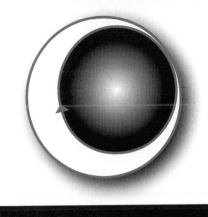

Core
Clinical
Cases in

Obstetrics and Gynaecology

Third edition

Gary Mires MBChB MD FRCOG FHEA
Professor of Obstetrics and Undergraduate Teaching
Dean, School of Medicine, Ninewells Hospital and
Medical School, University of Dundee, Dundee, UK

Khalid S. Khan MRCOG MSc MMEd
Professor of Women's Health and Clinical Epidemiology,
Institute of Health Sciences Education, Bart's and The
London School of Medicine and Dentistry, London, UK

Janesh K. Gupta MSc MD FRCOG
Professor in Obstetrics and Gynaecology, University
of Birmingham, Birmingham Women's Hospital,
Birmingham, UK

Core Clinical Cases series edited by

Janesh K. Gupta MSc MD FRCOG
Professor in Obstetrics and Gynaecology, University
of Birmingham, Birmingham Women's Hospital,
Birmingham, UK

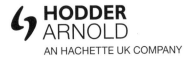
HODDER
ARNOLD
AN HACHETTE UK COMPANY

First published in Great Britain in 2001 by Arnold,
Second edition published in 2005 by Hodder Arnold
This third edition published in 2011 by Hodder Arnold, an imprint of Hodder
Education, a division of Hachette UK, 338 Euston Road, London NW1 3BH

http://www.hodderarnold.com

Whilst the advice and information in this book are believed to be true and accurate at the date
of going to press, neither the author[s] nor the publisher can accept any legal responsibility or
liability for any errors or omissions that may be made. In particular (but without limiting the
generality of the preceding disclaimer) every effort has been made to check drug dosages;
however it is still possible that errors have been missed. Furthermore, dosage schedules are
constantly being revised and new side effects recognized. For these reasons the reader is strongly
urged to consult the drug companies' printed instructions before administering any of the drugs
recommended in this book.

British Library Cataloguing in Publication Data
A catalogue record for this book is available from the British Library

Library of Congress Cataloging-in-Publication Data
A catalog record for this book is available from the Library of Congress

ISBN-13:   9781 4441 2285 5
2 3 4 5 6 7 8 9 10

Commissioning Editor: Joanna Koster
Project Editor: Stephen Clausard
Production Controller: Jonathan Williams
Cover Design: Amina Dudhia
Index: Merrall-Ross International Ltd

Typeset in Fruitiger 9/11 by MPS Limited, a Macmillan Company, Chennai
Printed and bound by CPI Group (UK) Ltd., Croydon, CR0 4YY

What do you think about this book? Or any other Hodder Arnold title?
Please visit our website: www.hodderarnold.com

Contents

Series preface
'A history lesson'

Between about 1916 and 1927 a puzzling illness appeared and swept around the world. Dr von Economo first described encephalitis lethargica (EL), which simply meant 'inflammation of the brain that makes you tired'. Younger people, especially women, seemed to be more vulnerable but the disease affected people of all ages. People with EL developed a 'sleep disorder', fever, headache and weakness, which led to a prolonged state of unconsciousness. The EL epidemic occurred during the same time period as the 1918 influenza pandemic, and the two outbreaks have been linked ever since in the medical literature. Some confused it with the epidemic of Spanish flu at that time whereas others blamed weapons used in World War I.

Encephalitis lethargica was dramatized by the film *Awakenings* (book written by Oliver Sacks, an eminent neurologist from New York), starring Robin Williams and Robert De Niro. Professor Sacks treated his patients with L-dopa, which temporarily awoke his patients, giving rise to the belief that the condition was related to Parkinson's disease.

Since the 1916–27 epidemic, only sporadic cases have been described. Pathological studies have revealed encephalitis of the midbrain and basal ganglia, with lymphocyte (predominantly plasma cell) infiltration. Recent examination of archived EL brain material has failed to demonstrate influenza RNA, adding to the evidence that EL was not invasive influenza encephalitis. Further investigations found no evidence of viral encephalitis or other recognized causes of rapid-onset parkinsonism. Magnetic resonance imaging of the brain was normal in 60 per cent but showed inflammatory changes localized to the deep grey matter in 40 per cent of patients.

As late as the end of twentieth century, it seemed that the possible answers lay in the clinical presentation of the patients in the 1916–27 epidemic. It had been noted by the clinicians, at that time, that the central nervous system (CNS) disorder had presented with pharyngitis. This led to the possibility of a post-infectious autoimmune CNS disorder similar to Sydenham's chorea, in which group A ß-haemolytic streptococcal antibodies cross-react with the basal ganglia and result in abnormal behaviour and involuntary movements. Anti-streptolysin-O titres have subsequently been found to be elevated in most of these patients. It seemed possible that autoimmune antibodies may cause remitting parkinsonian signs subsequent to streptococcal tonsillitis as part of the spectrum of post-streptococcal CNS disease.

Could it be that the 80-year mystery of EL has been solved relying on the patient's clinical history of presentation, rather than focusing on expensive investigations? More research in this area will give us the definitive answer. This scenario is not dissimilar to the controversy about the idea that streptococcal infections were aetiologically related to rheumatic fever.

With this example of a truly fascinating history lesson, we hope that you will endeavour to use the patient's clinical history as your most powerful diagnostic tool to make the correct diagnosis. If you do you are likely to be right between 80 and 90 per cent of the time. This is the basis of all the Core Clinical Cases series, which make you systematically explore clinical problems through the clinical history of presentation, followed by examination and then performing appropriate investigations. Never break those rules!

Janesh Gupta
2006

Preface

Why core clinical cases?

In undergraduate medical education there is a trend towards the development of 'core' curricula. The aim is to facilitate the teaching of essential and relevant knowledge, skills and attitudes. This is in sharp contrast to traditional curricula, where there was an emphasis on detailed factual information, often without any practical clinical relevance. Currently, students' learning is being more commonly examined using objective structured clinical examinations which assess the practical use of knowledge, rather than the regurgitation of small-print information that was commonly emphasized in traditional examination methods. This book has defined the 'core' material for obstetrics and gynaecology by considering the common core clinical problems which may be encountered in primary and secondary care, and it provides a learning strategy to master this 'core' material for examinations.

Why a problem-solving approach?

In practice, patients present with clinical problems, which are explored through history, examination and investigation, progressively leading from a differential to a definitive diagnosis. Unfortunately, standard textbooks tend to present the subject matter according to a pathophysiological classification that does not help to prepare students to confront clinical scenarios. We have therefore based this book on a problem-solving approach. This inculcates the capacity for critical thinking and helps students to analyse the basis of clinical problems. The deep understanding of learning issues acquired in this way means that knowledge can be more easily retrieved both to solve real patients' problems in the future and to answer confidently clinical questions encountered in examinations.

How will this book inspire problem-solving traits?

The short case scenarios presented in this book are based on common core clinical cases which students are likely to encounter in an undergraduate obstetrics and gynaecology module. We have grouped these cases according to areas of patients' complaints. There are seven groups in the gynaecology category and six groups in obstetrics. Each group includes five or six cases, which begin with a statement of the patient's complaint followed by a short description of the patient's problem. For each case, using a question and short answer format, the student is taken through a problem-solving exercise. There are two types of problem-solving cases in this book. One type deals with the development of a diagnostic and therapeutic strategy, and the other deals with the development of a counselling strategy. The sequence of the cases and questions in each patient's problem group is a logical one, taking the student from basics to the advanced aspects of clinical care. 'Core' information about the subject matter relevant to the patient's problem is also summarized, as this information is helpful for answering the questions. The format of the book enables the cases to be used for learning as well as for self-assessment.

In the cases that deal with diagnostic and therapeutic strategies, the student is questioned about the interpretation of all the relevant clinical features presented, in order to compile an array of likely differential diagnoses. They are then asked to identify specific pieces of information in the history and to select an appropriate clinical examination which will narrow down the differential list to the most likely diagnosis. This emphasis is important because, in clinical practice, history and examination alone result in a correct diagnosis in 80–90 per cent of patients. Following this, students are asked to suggest the investigations which would be required to confirm or refute the diagnosis. Once the diagnosis has been reached, students will develop a treatment plan. In general, this plan should first consider conservative non-invasive options (e.g. doing nothing), followed by medical and finally surgical options.

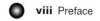

The therapeutic strategy will also have to be conveyed to the patient in a manner that he or she can understand. Therefore in each group, patient problems that will challenge students to develop a counselling strategy have been included. These counselling cases will help students to communicate confidently with patients (one counselling case has been included in the last chapter which gives an idea of the marking system that may be used in an examination situation). This generic learning strategy is followed throughout the book with the aim of reinforcing the skills required to master the problem-solving approach.

G. Mires
K. S. Khan
J. K. Gupta

Abbreviations used for investigations

✓	investigation required
±	optional investigation
✗	investigation not required
ßhCG	ß human chorionic gonadotrophin
AFI	amniotic fluid index
AFP	a-fetoprotein
ARM	artificial rupture of the membranes
BP	blood pressure
BPD	biparietal diameter
CHD	coronary heart disease
CIN	cervical intraepithelial neoplasia
COC	combined oral contraceptive pill
CRP	C-reactive protein
CT	computed tomography
CTG	cardiotocograph
D&C	dilatation and curettage
DIC	disseminated intravascular coagulation
DUB	dysfunctional uterine bleeding
DVT	deep vein thrombosis
EDD	estimated date of delivery
FAC	fetal abdominal circumference
FBC	full blood count
FHR	fetal heart rate
FSH	follicle-stimulating hormone
GnRH	gonadotrophin-releasing hormone
HELLP	haemolysis, elevated liver enzymes and low platelets
HPV	human papillomavirus
HRT	hormone replacement therapy
HSV	herpes simplex virus
HVS	high vaginal swab

ICSI	intracytoplasmic sperm injection
Ig	immunoglobulin
ITP	idiopathic thrombocytopenic purpura
IUCD	intrauterine contraceptive device
IUGR	intrauterine growth restriction
IVF	*in vitro* fertilization
IVF-ET	*in vitro* fertilization and embryo transfer
LBC	liquid-based cytology
LFD	large for dates
LFT	liver function test
LH	luteinizing hormone
LLETZ	large loop excision of the transformation zone
LMP	last menstrual period
MCH	mean cell haemoglobin
MCV	mean cell volume
MRI	magnetic resonance imaging
MSU	midstream specimen of urine
NSAID	non-steroidal anti-inflammatory drug
PCOS	polycystic ovarian syndrome
PID	pelvic inflammatory disease
PMB	postmenopausal bleeding
PMS	premenstrual syndrome
POP	progesterone-only pill
SGA	small for gestational age
SSRI	selective serotonin reuptake inhibitor
STI	sexually transmitted infection
TENS	transcutaneous electrical nerve stimulation
TFT	thyroid function test
TSH	thyroid-stimulating hormone
TTN	tachypnoea of the newborn
UA	umbilical artery
U&Es	urea and electrolytes
USS	ultrasound scan
UTI	urinary tract infection
WCC	white cell count

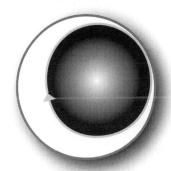

1 Early pregnancy problems

Questions

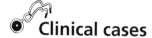 **Clinical cases**

For each of the case scenarios given, consider the following:

Q1: What is the likely differential diagnosis?
Q2: What issues in the given history support the diagnosis?
Q3: What additional features in the history would you seek to support a particular diagnosis?
Q4: What clinical examination would you perform and why?
Q5: What investigations would be most helpful and why?
Q6: What treatment options are appropriate?

CASE 1.1 – My period is 2 weeks late and I am bleeding.

A 23-year-old nulliparous woman has had 6 weeks of amenorrhoea. She has not been using any contraception. She normally has a regular menstrual cycle every 28 days. A pregnancy home test is positive. She has noticed slight vaginal spotting.

CASE 1.2 – I am 8 weeks pregnant and have pain and bleeding.

A 34-year-old woman presents with a history of 6 weeks of amenorrhoea, abdominal pain and slight vaginal bleeding. She stopped the oral contraceptive pill 2 years ago in order to conceive, and she recently booked an appointment to see her doctor because she was concerned that she was infertile. She has previously had an appendectomy and pelvic inflammatory disease (PID). Recently she has been feeling dizzy. A home pregnancy test is positive.

CASE 1.3 – I am pregnant and cannot keep anything down.

A 26-year-old primigravida presents at 8 weeks' gestation with a history of nausea and vomiting for the last 2 weeks. However, over the past 48h, she indicates that she has been unable to keep any food or drink down.

ᴀ̊ᴀ̊ OSCE counselling cases

OSCE COUNSELLING CASE 1.1 – **I am upset that my first pregnancy has ended in a miscarriage.**

A 23-year-old woman has had an evacuation of the uterus following an incomplete miscarriage at 10 weeks' gestation in her first pregnancy. She is ready for discharge home and very upset.

Q1: What counselling would you give her about miscarriage and about postoperative recovery before discharge?

OSCE COUNSELLING CASE 1.2 – **This is my third miscarriage. What can be done about it?**

A patient has just undergone an evacuation of the uterus for her third consecutive spontaneous miscarriage. She has had no pregnancies beyond 10 weeks' gestation.

Q1: What investigations should be undertaken?

Q2: In the absence of any identifiable cause, what are her chances of achieving an ongoing pregnancy on the next occasion?

🔑 Key concepts

In order to work through the core clinical cases in this chapter, you will need to understand the following key concepts.

BLEEDING IN EARLY PREGNANCY

- Bleeding in early pregnancy is very common.
- 20 per cent of pregnancies undergo spontaneous miscarriage.
- Ectopic pregnancy should be considered in the differential diagnosis in all women of reproductive age presenting with abdominal pain and vaginal bleeding.

Answers

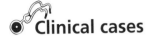 **Clinical cases**

CASE 1.1 – **My period is 2 weeks late and I am bleeding.**

A1: What is the likely differential diagnosis?

- Miscarriage
  - threatened miscarriage;
  - inevitable miscarriage;
  - incomplete miscarriage;
  - complete miscarriage;
  - missed miscarriage.
- Ectopic pregnancy (see Case 1.2).
- Molar pregnancy.

A2: What issues in the given history support the diagnosis?

Six weeks of amenorrhoea and a positive pregnancy test, after regular menstrual cycles, indicate an early pregnancy. The small amount of bleeding is a sign that the patient is threatening to have a miscarriage. However, a firm diagnosis can be established only after further investigations.

A3: What additional features in the history would you seek to support a particular diagnosis?

The degree of bleeding, associated pain and passage of products of conception would indicate the type of miscarriage (Table 1.1).

A4: What clinical examination would you perform and why?

Assess the patient's haemodynamic status, including blood pressure (hypotension in hypovolaemic shock), pulse (tachycardia in hypovolaemic shock) and degree of bleeding. The temperature should be taken to exclude infection in septic miscarriage. An abdominal examination is essential to elicit signs of rebound tenderness and acute abdomen (ectopic pregnancy).

Speculum examination should be performed to visualize the cervical os and determine whether fetal tissue is present in the os or the vagina. The nature of the cervical os (open/closed) on digital examination will help to distinguish between the different types of miscarriage (see Table 1.1). Uterine size should be assessed during bimanual examination. Uterine tenderness is unlikely unless there is septic miscarriage. Vaginal examination may elicit cervical excitation (pelvic tenderness on moving the cervix) and adnexal tenderness in ectopic pregnancy.

A5: What investigations would be most helpful and why?

• **Urine ßhCG**	✓	To confirm pregnancy. Home pregnancy tests may be unreliable.
• **FBC**	✓	To assess blood loss and measure white cell count (WCC) and differential as a marker of infection.

Table 1.1 Summary of key features in the history, examination, investigations and outcome for the various types of miscarriage and ectopic pregnancy

Type of miscarriage	History — Pain	Examination — Bleeding	Examination — Cervical os	Investigation — Uterine size in relation to gestational age	Investigation — Uterus on ultrasound scan	Management/outcome
Threatened	Slight/none	Slight to moderate	Closed	Consistent	Fetus with heart beat	Approx. 25 per cent will miscarry
Inevitable	Moderate	Moderate/heavy	Open	Small or consistent	Fetus may be alive	Miscarriage is inevitable
Incomplete	Moderate	Heavy, some fetal tissue parts may have been passed	Open	Small	Some fetal tissue	Will need evacuation of uterus by medical/surgical means
Complete	Slight at presentation, but moderate earlier on	Slight to moderate after heavier loss	Initially open, then closed after miscarriage	Small	Empty	No treatment required
Missed	Absent	None/slight	Closed	Consistent or small	Fetus with no heart beat	Will need evacuation of uterus by medical/surgical means
Septic	Moderate	Moderate/offensive	Open	Consistent or small	Empty or fetal tissue	Antibiotics and evacuation of retained products of conception
Molar	Slight/none	Slight to moderate	Closed	Consistent or large	Classic 'snowstorm' appearance of vesicles	Will need surgical evacuation of uterus and follow-up
Ectopic	Variable: none to moderate/severe	None/slight	Closed/cervical excitation	Small	Empty uterus	See Case 1.2

- **CRP** ☑ If temperature is elevated or there are other signs of infection, e.g. offensive vaginal loss.

- **Blood group** ± To check rhesus status and administer anti-D if indicated (see Revision panel, p.12).

- **Group and save, cross-match** ☑ In cases of shock.

- **USS** ☑ To determine whether the fetus is intrauterine and if it is viable. It will also detect retained fetal tissue (products of conception). The absence of intrauterine fetal tissue (i.e. empty uterus) should suggest the possibility of an ectopic pregnancy.

- **Serum ßhCG** ☑ There is a doubling of levels within 48h in a viable intrauterine pregnancy.

- **Histology** ☑ Any tissue expelled from the uterus should be sent for histology to exclude molar pregnancy. Sometimes the tissue is an endometrial cast without any trophoblast, indicating an ectopic pregnancy.

A6: What treatment options are appropriate?

CONSERVATIVE

Bedrest does not prevent miscarriage. Admission to hospital in cases of threatened miscarriage is not always necessary.

MEDICAL

Intramuscular ergometrine may be required to reduce heavy bleeding in cases of incomplete, inevitable or complete miscarriage. In patients with mild bleeding, it may be possible to avoid surgical evacuation in incomplete miscarriage by using mifepristone and prostaglandins to induce evacuation of the uterus. The patient should be warned of prolonged irregular bleeding.

SURGICAL

- Removal of fetal tissue from the os can stop uncontrollable bleeding. In incomplete or missed miscarriage, evacuation of retained products of conception under general anaesthetic is used to prevent continued bleeding and risk of infection.
- Antibiotics are required if there is evidence of suspected or confirmed infection.

CASE 1.2 – I am 8 weeks pregnant and have pain and bleeding.

A1: What is the likely differential diagnosis?

- Ectopic pregnancy.
- Miscarriage (see Case 1.1).

A2: What issues in the given history support the diagnosis?

Diagnosis of ectopic pregnancy can be difficult. A period of amenorrhoea, abdominal/pelvic pain and slight bleeding is classically associated with ectopic pregnancy. Syncopal episodes (fainting/dizziness) are associated with fallopian tube distension and stimulation of the autonomic nervous system. Previous surgery (e.g. appendectomy), PID and conception after infertility are all risk factors for ectopic pregnancy.

A3: What additional features in the history would you seek to support a particular diagnosis?

Any factors that may damage the fallopian tubes are risk factors for ectopic pregnancy, including PID secondary to a sexually transmitted infection (STI) or an intrauterine contraceptive device (IUCD). Tubal surgery, such as reversal of sterilization and salpingostomy for hydrosalpinges, and assisted conception (e.g. *in vitro* fertilization or IVF) are additional risk factors. Other symptoms include shoulder-tip pain resulting from irritation of the diaphragm by blood leaking from the ectopic.

A4: What clinical examination would you perform and why?

Assessment of the patient's haemodynamic status by checking blood pressure (to detect hypotension) and pulse (to detect tachycardia) will indicate the degree of blood loss. An abdominal examination should be performed to elicit tenderness to palpation, rebound tenderness, guarding or rigidity, as well as gentle vaginal examination to detect cervical excitation (pelvic tenderness on moving the cervix) and the possibility of palpating a tender adnexal mass. Care should be taken not to convert an unruptured stable ectopic to an emergency situation by compressing and rupturing an ectopic mass during bimanual vaginal examination. This examination should therefore not be undertaken in a community setting.

A5: What investigations would be most helpful and why?

- **Urine ßhCG** ✓ This should always be tested in women of reproductive age, who present with pain and bleeding, to confirm pregnancy.

- **FBC** ✓ To assess the systemic effect of bleeding and measure WCC and differential as a marker of infection.

- **CRP** ✓ If temperature elevated or other signs of infection, e.g. offensive vaginal loss.

- **Blood group** ✓ To check the patient's rhesus status and administer anti-D if indicated (see Revision panel, p. 12).

- **Group and save, cross-match** ✓ In cases of shock.

- **Serum ßhCG** ✓ Normally, a doubling of levels in 48 h is associated with intrauterine pregnancy. This test should be undertaken if conservative management is planned in a stable patient.

- **USS (preferably transvaginal)** ✓ This can indicate an intrauterine pregnancy as early as 6 weeks' amenorrhoea. An empty uterus, fluid in the pouch of Douglas and an adnexal mass on USS would give a high index of suspicion of ectopic pregnancy.

- **Diagnostic laparoscopy** ✓ This is the gold standard for confirming the diagnosis. Very early ectopics can still be missed at laparoscopy. The false-negative rate is about 5 per cent.

A6: What treatment options are appropriate?

CONSERVATIVE

- There is no place for conservative management in ectopic pregnancy if the patient is *symptomatic*, because this is a life-threatening condition. The patient should be admitted to hospital and definitive treatment administered.

- A conservative approach would be appropriate only if the patient was asymptomatic and, after investigations, there was uncertainty about the diagnosis. A very early intrauterine pregnancy may not be visible on a scan, but serum ßhCG repeated after 48 h would show a doubling of levels if the pregnancy was viable. If the pregnancy is not viable, ßhCG levels will fall and will eventually become undetectable.

MEDICAL

Unruptured ectopics less than 3–4 cm in size can be treated with methotrexate systemically or by administering it into the ectopic sac under USS or laparoscopic guidance. Follow-up with ßhCG is essential because the risk of persistent ectopic pregnancy is high. This method may allow the tube to function in the future, because 60 per cent of women will subsequently have a successful pregnancy. There is a 15 per cent risk of recurrent ectopic pregnancy.

SURGICAL

This may involve laparoscopy or laparotomy.
- Milking of the ectopic or salpingotomy can be used for removal of an ectopic pregnancy without removing the tube. Both of these procedures salvage the tube, but follow-up with ßhCG is essential to exclude a persistent ectopic pregnancy.
- Salpingectomy involves removal of the ectopic with the tube. Follow-up with ßhCG is not necessary in this case.

CASE 1.3 – I am pregnant and cannot keep anything down.

A1: What is the likely differential diagnosis?
- Hyperemesis gravidarum.
- Urinary tract infection (UTI).
- Appendicitis.
- Gastrointestinal infection.
- Rarer problems (e.g. bowel obstruction, hepatic disorders or cerebral tumours).

A2: What issues in the given history support the diagnosis?

Pregnancy and vomiting of all food and drink support the diagnosis of hyperemesis, particularly in the first trimester.

A3: What additional features in the history would you seek to support a particular diagnosis?

Acute onset of the problem would support a diagnosis such as gastroenteritis or appendicitis. A longer duration of the symptoms with pre-existing nausea/vomiting would support a diagnosis of hyperemesis. Associated symptoms (e.g. diarrhoea, urinary symptoms, abdominal pain), other members of the family with the same problem or symptoms of thyrotoxicosis would support a diagnosis other than hyperemesis.

A4: What clinical examination would you perform and why?

Look for evidence of dehydration (e.g. dry mouth, tachycardia or postural hypotension). Abdominal signs of tenderness and guarding would support a diagnosis of appendicitis. A large-for-dates uterus may suggest multiple pregnancy as a cause of hyperemesis.

A5: What investigations would be most helpful and why?

- **FBC**   ☑   Haemoglobin for haemoconcentration and WCC for infection.

- **U&Es**   ☑   To check for dehydration.

- **Urinalysis**   ☑   The presence of ketones supports a history of excessive vomiting. The presence of leucocytes and/or protein supports a diagnosis of urinary tract infection (UTI).

- **MSU**   ☑   To exclude UTI.

- **USS**   ☑   To exclude molar and multiple pregnancy. Hyperemesis is more common in these cases. Trisomy 18, features and/or markers for which can be seen on ultrasound, can cause prolonged severe vomiting extending into the late second trimester.

- **LFT**   ±   For liver disorders.

- **TSH**   ±   To exclude thyrotoxicosis. Note that thyroid-stimulating hormone (TSH) can be suppressed in hyperemesis.

- **Stool sample**   ±   If diarrhoea is present for more than 48h.

A6: What treatment options are appropriate?

Conditions other than hyperemesis require treatment specific to the problem (e.g. evacuate molar pregnancy with appropriate follow-up (urinary and serum ßhCG and avoiding pregnancy with adequate contraception until normal ßhCG has been obtained; appendectomy for appendicitis; antibiotics for UTI).

HYPEREMESIS

- Supportive:
  - admit the patient to hospital;
  - reassure her that this problem is likely to resolve spontaneously at 12–14 weeks;
  - offer psychological support (many women have additional social and emotional problems).
- Medical:
  - intravenous fluids – 24/48h to clear ketones and rehydrate;
  - antiemetics (prochlorperazine, intramuscular or suppository; intramuscular metoclopramide; intravenous ondansetron; oral when vomiting settled);
  - introduce foods as appropriate in small amounts – avoid fatty foods;
  - steroids may be given in severe cases;
  - vitamin supplementation (vitamin B_6, if prolonged vomiting occurs);
  - may occasionally require parenteral nutrition.
- Surgical:
  - in severe cases, termination of pregnancy may need to be considered.

👥 OSCE counselling cases

OSCE COUNSELLING CASE 1.1 – **I am upset that my first pregnancy has ended in a miscarriage.**

A1: What counselling would you give her about miscarriage and about postoperative recovery before discharge?

MISCARRIAGE

Miscarriage is very common, with approximately one in five pregnancies ending in miscarriage.
- Most are unexplained.
- There is nothing that the patient could have done that would have caused the miscarriage.
- There is nothing that she could have done to prevent the miscarriage.
- Her risk of miscarriage in the next pregnancy is not increased.

POSTOPERATIVE RECOVERY

- The patient can expect some continued vaginal blood loss for a few days. It should not be heavy or offensive, and should gradually tail off. If the loss becomes heavy and fresh or offensive, she should seek medical help.
- There is no medical reason why she needs to delay further attempts at pregnancy, but she must feel psychologically ready. You might suggest waiting for one normal period.
- If she needs additional support, offer her contact telephone numbers and information about early pregnancy loss support groups within the local area. In addition, you might offer a follow-up appointment if she would find this helpful.
- If she is rhesus negative, and she meets the requirements for administration, ensure that she has had anti-D before discharge and explain the reasons for this.

OSCE COUNSELLING CASE 1.2 – **This is my third miscarriage. What can be done about it?**

A1: What investigations should be undertaken?

- Three consecutive miscarriages are defined as recurrent miscarriage. This is more often associated with an identifiable cause than are isolated cases of miscarriage.
- Investigations would include the following:
  - chromosomal analysis of the products of conception;
  - chromosomal analysis of both parents – a chromosomal abnormality (e.g. balanced translocation) will be diagnosed in one of the partners in 3–5 per cent of cases of recurrent miscarriage;
  - maternal blood for anticardiolipin antibodies and lupus anticoagulant to exclude antiphospholipid syndrome present in 15 per cent of cases of recurrent miscarriage;
  - a pelvic ultrasound to assess uterine anatomy and morphology.

A2: In the absence of any identifiable cause, what are her chances of achieving an ongoing pregnancy on the next occasion?

There is a 60–70 per cent likelihood of successful pregnancy if no cause is found for recurrent miscarriage.

REVISION PANEL

Rhesus prophylaxis following early pregnancy loss:
- Not all RhD negative women require anti-D immunoglobulin following early pregnancy loss.

The following is taken from Royal College of Obstetricians and Gynaecologists Greentop Guideline 22. The Use of Anti-D Immunoglobulin for Rhesus D Prophylaxis and gives a guide to those who do.
- *Ectopic pregnancy*: Anti-D Ig should be given to all non-sensitized RhD negative women who have an ectopic pregnancy.
- *Spontaneous miscarriage*: Anti-D Ig should be given to all non-sensitized RhD negative women who have a spontaneous complete or incomplete abortion after 12 weeks of pregnancy. Anti-D Ig should be given to such women prior to 12 weeks when there has been an intervention to evacuate the uterus.
- *Threatened miscarriage*: Anti-D Ig should be given to all non-sensitized RhD negative women with a threatened miscarriage after 12 weeks of pregnancy. Where bleeding continues intermittently after 12 weeks' gestation, anti-D Ig should be given at 6-weekly intervals. Routine administration of anti-D Ig in threatened miscarriage before 12 weeks is not recommended. However it may be prudent to administer anti-D Ig where bleeding is heavy or repeated or where there is associated abdominal pain, particularly if these events occur as gestation approaches 12 weeks.

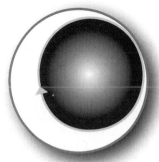

2 Pregnancy dating and fetal growth

Questions

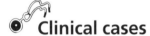

Clinical cases

For each of the case scenarios given, consider the following:

Q1: What is the likely differential diagnosis?
Q2: What issues in the given history support the diagnosis?
Q3: What additional features in the history would you seek to support a particular diagnosis?
Q4: What clinical examination would you perform and why?
Q5: What investigations would be most helpful and why?
Q6: What treatment options are appropriate?

CASE 2.1 – I think I am pregnant, but I cannot remember the date of my last menstrual period.

A 23-year-old woman has a positive pregnancy test but is uncertain about the exact stage of her pregnancy. She thinks that her last period was 4 months ago. She has had irregular and infrequent periods in the past. She has presented for her first antenatal visit, in her first pregnancy.

CASE 2.2 – The midwife says my baby is small.

A 28-year-old in her second pregnancy attends the midwife antenatal clinic at 32 weeks' gestation. There are adequate fetal movements, but the midwife is concerned that the uterus feels small for dates. The symphysiofundal height is 27 cm. The patient admits to smoking 20 cigarettes per day. Her antenatal care to date has been uneventful.

CASE 2.3 – The midwife says my baby is big.

A 32-year-old woman in her third pregnancy attends the midwife antenatal clinic at 34 weeks' gestation. The midwife is concerned that the uterus feels large for dates. A booking scan had shown a singleton pregnancy consistent with menstrual dates. The symphysiofundal height measures 40 cm. There were no anomalies noted on her 20-week scan. The patient has experienced increasing abdominal discomfort during the last 2 weeks, and she is having irregular uterine activity. In addition, she has noticed an increase in shortness of breath.

👫 OSCE counselling cases

OSCE COUNSELLING CASE 2.1 – **I have been told that my baby is small. How am I going to be monitored?**

A woman in her first pregnancy attends the antenatal clinic at 34 weeks. On examination, the uterus feels small for dates, and an ultrasound scan (USS) confirms that the abdominal circumference is below the fifth centile for gestation. The liquor volume is reported to be within normal limits, and the umbilical Doppler ultrasound is normal. The woman reports that the baby is active.

Q1: Counsel this patient about the findings and how you propose to monitor fetal well-being.

OSCE COUNSELLING CASE 2.2 – **I want to have screening for Down's syndrome. What is involved?**

A 24-year-old primigravida at 10 weeks' gestation attends the antenatal clinic. She has read about testing for Down's syndrome in a magazine and wishes to discuss this with you.

Q1: Counsel her about screening for Down's syndrome.

⚷ Key concepts

In order to work through the core clinical cases in this chapter, you will need to understand the following key concepts.

SMALL FOR GESTATIONAL AGE (SGA)

Term used to describe a fetus with a birthweight <10th centile corrected for gestation, sex of baby, maternal height and weight, ethnic origin and birth order. This may reflect:
- A fetus that has grown normally but is constitutionally small

or
- Chronic compromise resulting from 'placental insufficiency', leading to intrauterine growth restriction (IUGR).

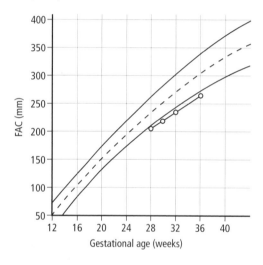

Figure 2.1 Fetal abdominal circumference (FAC) in a small-for-gestational-age (SGA) fetus with normal growth (constitutionally small). The FAC is increasing with gestation at an appropriate rate, i.e. parallel to the centile line but <5th centile.

INTRAUTERINE GROWTH RESTRICTION

The fetus is failing to achieve its growth potential (e.g. if a fetus is genetically determined to be 3.8 kg but only achieves 2.8 kg).

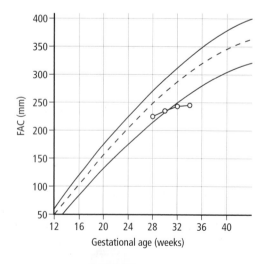

Figure 2.2 Fetal abdominal circumference (FAC) in a small-for-gestational-age (SGA) fetus with abnormal growth (intrauterine growth restriction or IUGR). The FAC crosses the centile line with increasing gestation, i.e. at 28 weeks above the 5th centile line but at 34 weeks well below the 5th centile line.

VIABILITY

Taken to be after 24 completed weeks in the UK.

LARGE FOR DATES

Term used to describe a fetus with a corrected birthweight >95th centile for gestational age.

MACROSOMIA

Birthweight >4.5 kg.

POLYHYDRAMNIOS

Excess amniotic fluid (>8 cm average liquor pocket depth or an amniotic fluid index (AFI: sum of pocket depths of liquor in four uterine quadrants) >25 on ultrasound, but is dependent on gestational age).

OLIGOHYDRAMNIOS

Reduced amniotic fluid (<2 cm average liquor pocket depth or an AFI <5 on ultrasound).

TERM

Pregnancy between 37 and 42 completed gestational weeks.

PRE-TERM

Pregnancy before 37 completed gestational weeks.

POST-TERM

Pregnancy beyond 42 completed gestational weeks.

GRAVIDA

Number of pregnancies, including current pregnancy.

PARITY

Two values are given. The first is the number of pregnancies beyond 24 weeks plus those ending before 24 weeks in which there were signs of life, and the second is the number of pregnancies ending before 24 weeks without signs of life.

Box 2.1 Cardiotocography

Components of a cardiotocograph (CTG)

A CTG is a combined pictorial representation of the continuous recording made up of two components:
- '*Cardio*' component: fetal heart trace measured by external ultrasound Sonicaid, or by an electrode attached to the fetal scalp (or fetal buttock) during labour.
- *Toco*' component: measurement of uterine contraction activity assessed by external strain gauge transducer.
- The *normal* recommended paper speed should be set at 1 cm/min to allow for correct interpretation.

Reasons why a CTG is performed

- During the antenatal period, a 'non-stress test' (when no contractions are expected) by a CTG is a method of assessing fetal well-being.
- During the intrapartum period, continuous recording is used to detect 'fetal distress', with the aim of detecting fetal hypoxia.

Features of a normal CTG (Fig. 2.3)

- The baseline rate can range from 110 to 160 beats/min for a term fetus.
- The 'beat-to-beat' baseline variability should be >5 beats/min.
- There are no decelerations.
- There are at least two accelerations (>15 beats/min for 15 s) in a 20-min trace often in response to fetal movements. This indicates a healthy 'reactive' trace.

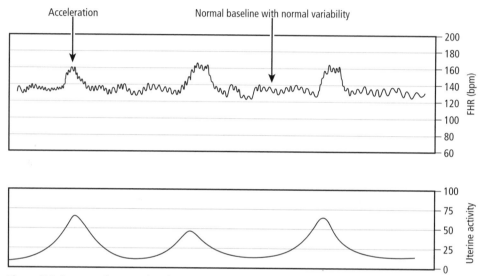

Figure 2.3 Features of a normal cardiotocograph.

Types of abnormalities that a CTG can detect

- Early deceleration: deceleration beginning with the onset of the contraction, returning to the baseline rate by the end of the contraction. Usually caused by head compression as the cervix dilates over the wide anterior fontanelle, but can result from cord compression or early hypoxia (Fig. 2.4).

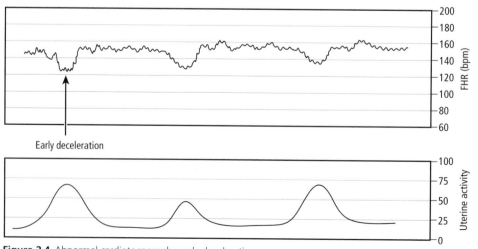

Figure 2.4 Abnormal cardiotocograph: early decelerations.

- Variable deceleration: deceleration appearing at a variable time during the contraction, of irregular shape, >15 beats/min and lasting for at least 15 s but <2 min. They are often caused by cord compression.

- Late deceleration: deceleration trough is the lowest point, which is past the peak of the contraction (the lag time). Late decelerations are associated with fetal hypoxia. The most worrying CTG is one that has a combination of loss of beat-to-beat variability, fetal tachycardia and late decelerations. This appearance is strongly associated with fetal hypoxia (about 60 per cent of cases) (Fig. 2.5).

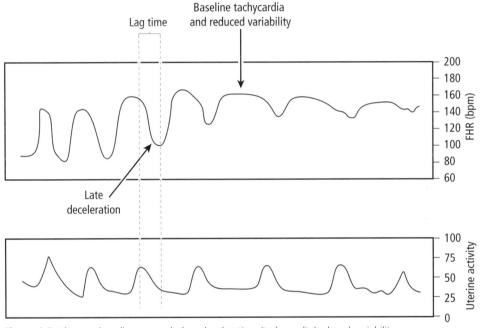

Figure 2.5 Abnormal cardiotocograph: late decelerations/tachycardia/reduced variability.

CTGs are usually classified as reassuring, non-reassuring or abnormal. The criteria for classification are given in Table 2.1.

Table 2.1 Classification of CTGs

Feature	Baseline (bpm)	Variability (bpm)	Decelerations	Accelerations
Reassuring	110–60	≥5	None	Present
Non-reassuring	100–9	<5 for 40–90 min	Typical variable decelerations with over 50 per cent of contractions, occurring for over 90 min	The absence of accelerations with otherwise normal trace is of uncertain significance
	161–80		Single prolonged deceleration for up to 3 min	
Abnormal	<100	<5 for >90 min	Either atypical variable decelerations with over 50 per cent of contractions or late decelerations, both for over 30 min	
	>180	Sinusoidal pattern ≥10 min	Single prolonged deceleration for more than 3 min	

National Institute of Health and Clinical Excellence. *Intrapartum care: care of healthy women and their babies during childbirth*. Clinical guideline 55. London: NICE, 2007.

Another approach to assessing fetal well-being is the biophysical profile. This is a 30-min USS which considers amniotic fluid (liquor) volume, fetal tone, fetal breathing movements and fetal movements in addition to a CTG. The scoring criteria are shown in Table 2.2.

Table 2.2 Biophysical profiles: scoring criteria

Biophysical variable	Normal (score 2)	Abnormal (score 0)
Fetal breathing movements	>1 episode for 30 s in 30 min	Absent/<30 s in 30 min
Gross body movements	>3 body/limb movements in 30 min	<3 body/limb movements in 30 min
Fetal tone	>1 episode body/limb extension followed by return	Slow, or absent extension–flexion of body or limbs to flexion, open–close cycle of fetal hand
Reactive fetal heart rate	>2 accelerations with fetal movements in 30 min	<2 accelerations, or 1+ deceleration in 30 min
Qualitative amniotic fluid	>1 pool of fluid, at least 1 cm × 1 cm	Either no measurable pool, or a pool <1 cm × 1 cm

A score of 8 or 10 suggests that the fetus is in good condition, a fetus scoring 6 may be 'sleeping' and a repeat biophysical profile later the same day should be performed, and a score of 0, 2 or 4 suggests that fetal compromise and delivery should be considered.

Answers

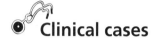

Clinical cases

CASE 2.1 – I think I am pregnant, but I cannot remember the date of my last menstrual period.

A1: What is the likely differential diagnosis?

Uncertain dates – pregnancy dating is crucial in this patient's further management because prenatal biochemical screening for Down's syndrome is dependent on gestational age. Furthermore, decisions about the type and frequency of antenatal care, as well as decisions about delivery, particularly post-term delivery, are also dependent on pregnancy dating.

A2: What issues in the given history support the diagnosis?

The irregular infrequent periods support the dating uncertainty. The first day of the last menstrual period (LMP) is usually used to calculate the estimated date of delivery (EDD) (e.g. by the obstetric 'wheel'). This is only accurate if there is a regular 28-day cycle, assuming that ovulation occurs 14 days before the next menstrual period. A longer cycle would require an upward adjustment of the EDD by the number of days that the cycle is longer than 28 days (e.g. adding 7 days if the cycle length is 35 days). This, along with uncertainty of LMP, makes an attempt at dating the pregnancy by this method inaccurate.

A3: What additional features in the history would you seek to support a particular diagnosis?

A detailed menstrual history should be obtained, as well as a history of contraceptive use (e.g. recent use of the combined pill or Depo-Provera, which may make ovulation timing unpredictable after cessation of contraception).

A4: What clinical examination would you perform and why?

- General health and nutritional status (gestational diabetes is more common in overweight women).
- Height (dystocia is more common in short [<150 cm] women).
- Baseline blood pressure.
- Chest examination (to identify previously undiagnosed heart murmurs).
- Breast examination (to detect incidental breast disease).
- The patient's abdomen should be palpated in order to determine the pregnancy size. The uterus is usually palpable abdominally at 12–14 weeks' gestation. The fundus reaches the umbilicus at 20 weeks' gestation. Thereafter, each additional gestational week is measured as a 1-cm increase in the symphysiofundal height (Fig. 2.6).

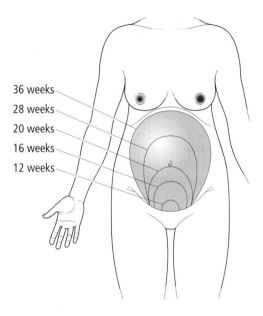

36 weeks
28 weeks
20 weeks
16 weeks
12 weeks

Figure 2.6 Uterine size in pregnancy.

A5: What investigations would be most helpful and why?

● **Urinalysis**	✓	To exclude proteinuria, which may indicate an asymptomatic urinary tract infection (UTI). Also glycosuria which may indicate gestational or undiagnosed type 2 diabetes.
● **Urine culture**	✓	Asymptomatic bacteriuria can lead to pyelonephritis.
● **FBC**	✓	To exclude anaemia.
● **Rhesus and antibody screen**	✓	If rhesus negative will need to be offered antenatal anti-D prophylaxis at 28 and 34 weeks.
● **Timed plasma glucose**	✓	To exclude gestational or undiagnosed type 2 diabetes, the incidence of which is increasing. Note that gestational diabetes in early gestation is rare and most cases diagnosed at this stage will be type 2. However, by definition any diagnosis of diabetes in pregnancy is gestational.
● **Serology for syphilis**	✓	
● **Rubella IgG**	✓	If not immune will be offered immunization in the postnatal period.
● **USS**	✓	A USS is mandatory in this case, and would be the most accurate way of dating this pregnancy. The fetal crown–rump length is an accurate measurement up to 12 weeks' gestation.

The biparietal diameter (BPD) is used between 14 and 20 weeks. After 20 weeks, growth patterns differ between fetuses, and there is no accurate measurement that reflects gestational age. Other advantages of ultrasound are exclusion of multiple pregnancies, maternal reassurance and detection of fetal structural abnormalities.

Consider:
- Down's syndrome screening.
- HIV and hepatitis B and C screening.
- Haemoglobin electrophoresis for at-risk individuals (e.g. those from the Mediterranean region and Asia).

A6: What treatment options are appropriate?

Subsequent antenatal care should be provided as for a normal pregnancy.

CASE 2.2 – The midwife says my baby is small.

A1: What is the likely differential diagnosis?

- Small for gestational age: normally growing but constitutionally small fetus.
- Intrauterine growth restriction.
- Wrong dates and the fetus is an appropriate size for the correct gestation.

A2: What issues in the given history support the diagnosis?

The uterus measurement being small for dates supports SGA or IUGR. Heavy smoking is associated with IUGR.

A3: What additional features in the history would you seek to support a particular diagnosis?

Checking the certainty of the patient's dates is essential (i.e. accuracy of menstrual data, and findings on USSs in the first and early second [up to 20 weeks] trimester). This is because, if the pregnancy is not as advanced as is believed, this could explain the discrepancy between the symphysiofundal height and gestational age. Additional risk factors for IUGR are a previous small-for-dates baby, maternal illness (e.g. hypertension), maternal infection in pregnancy (e.g. rubella, cytomegalovirus), and history of antepartum haemorrhage.

A4: What clinical examination would you perform and why?

Examination would include blood pressure measurement to exclude hypertension and pre-eclampsia, which are both associated with IUGR. A clinical assessment of liquor volume should be made because IUGR can be associated with reduced liquor volume. The fetal heart should be auscultated and a CTG performed because fetal compromise and intrauterine death are associated with IUGR.

A5: What investigations would be most helpful and why?

• **Urinalysis**	✓	Proteinuria indicates pre-eclampsia if blood pressure is high.
• **Cardiotocography**	✓	To identify evidence of fetal compromise.

- **USS** ✓   This should be performed (1) to measure abdominal circumference and BPD in order to confirm SGA, (2) to assess liquor volume, (3) to perform umbilical arterial (UA), middle cerebral artery (MCA) and ductus venosus (DV) Doppler assessment if SGA confirmed and (4) to perform a biophysical profile. Ultrasound may also indicate features of congenital infection (brain calcification) or structural anomaly (cardiac defect). UA Doppler is an indicator of placental resistance and hence indirectly placental function. Abnormal MCA and DV Doppler is an indicator that redistribution of the fetal circulation has occurred and hence hypoxia is likely, i.e. in hypoxia the fetus redistributes blood to the brain.

- **Amniocentesis or chorionic villus sample** ±   This may be considered if there are features on the USS that support a chromosomal anomaly or if severe early onset IUGR is identified. This can be associated with a chromosomal anomaly.

- **Fetal blood sample (cordocentesis)** ±   This is performed only in fetal medicine centres. It may be useful if congenital infection is suspected.

A6: What treatment options are appropriate?

The mainstay of management is to deliver a fetus as mature and in as good a condition as possible.

- Serial ultrasound examination should be performed to monitor the velocity of fetal growth in order to distinguish between a constitutionally small fetus and an IUGR fetus. The fetus that is growing and not showing evidence of compromise does not require any intervention.
- Umbilical Doppler waveform patterns in association with middle cerebral artery and ductus venosus Doppler, which if abnormal suggest redistribution of fetal blood supply and biophysical assessment, including cardiotocography, are required to identify evidence of fetal compromise.
- Specific aetiological conditions need appropriate management (e.g. hypertension).
- Steroids to promote surfactant production and reduce the risk or severity of respiratory distress syndrome in the case of pre-term delivery.

Box 2.2 Risks of intrauterine growth restriction and small for gestational age

Antepartum:
- hypoxia;
- intrauterine death.

Peripartum:
- hypoxia;
- intrauterine death;
- meconium aspiration.

Postpartum:
- neonatal hypoglycaemia;
- hypocalcaemia;
- hypothermia;
- polycythaemia;
- hypoxic–ischaemic encephalopathy;
- hypoxia during the antenatal and intrapartum period can result in developmental delay and cerebral palsy.

CASE 2.3 – **The midwife says my baby is big.**

A1: What is the likely differential diagnosis?
- Constitutionally large for dates (LFD).
- Macrosomia (e.g. secondary to diabetes).
- Wrong dates.
- Polyhydramnios.
- Multiple pregnancy.
- Hydrops.

A2: What issues in the given history support the diagnosis?
The uterus is clinically LFD based on symphysiofundal height. The increased discomfort, irritable uterus and shortness of breath suggest polyhydramnios. The previous dating and second-trimester USSs have excluded multiple pregnancy and fetal anomaly which might be associated with polyhydramnios (e.g. duodenal atresia).

A3: What additional features in the history would you seek to support a particular diagnosis?
A family history (e.g. first-degree relative with diabetes) or maternal obesity increases the risk of gestational diabetes and macrosomia.

Previous high birthweights would support a fetus that is constitutionally LFD. Rhesus factor and antibody checks are needed to exclude rhesus isoimmunization, which may be associated with fetal hydrops.

A4: What clinical examination would you perform and why?
Abdominal palpation is necessary to assess liquor volume. A tense uterus, difficulty in feeling fetal parts and fluid thrill all support an increased liquor volume.

A5: What investigations would be most helpful and why?
- **Glucose tolerance test (GTT)**   ✓   Fasting level >5.1 mmol/L and 2 h level >8.5 mmol/L would support a diagnosis of gestational diabetes.

- **USS**   ✓   To:
  - confirm LFD (BPD, abdominal circumference);
  - measure liquor volume;
  - exclude multiple pregnancy;
  - exclude fetal anomaly that may have been missed on earlier scans (fetal micturition and swallowing mechanisms are essential to maintain normal liquor volume; gut

atresia and neurological abnormalities such as anencephaly are associated with polyhydramnios because liquor cannot be swallowed);
- identify evidence of hydrops (e.g. fetal oedema/pleural effusions and/or ascites). If present look at fetal heart to exclude congenital cardiac defect.

- **Rhesus status and antibodies**   ☑   To exclude rhesus isoimmunization.

- **Erythrovirus B19 serology**   ±   If evidence of hydrops.

A6: What treatment options are appropriate?

If constitutionally LFD no action is required. This is not an indication for induction of labour or caesarean section.
- If gestational diabetes is diagnosed, it should be managed in a multidisciplinary clinic with dietary control and oral hypoglycaemic agent/insulin if blood sugars not controlled with an appropriate diet (preprandial less than 7 mmol/L).
- Polyhydramnios without symptoms and evidence of fetal anomaly does not require any treatment. In cases near term where there is maternal discomfort, induction of labour should be considered.
  - In cases where the fetus is premature and maternal discomfort is a problem, serial amniocentesis may be considered. However, there is a risk of pre-term labour and infection, and the fluid rapidly reaccumulates;
  - Indometacin can reduce liquor volume, but the risk to the fetus is premature closure of the ductus arteriosus and reduced cerebral perfusion;
  - As pre-term delivery is a risk, two doses of steroids (betamethasone 12 mg), 12 h apart, should be given to the mother to promote lung maturity and reduce the risk of respiratory distress syndrome.

♟♟ OSCE counselling cases

OSCE COUNSELLING CASE 2.1 – I have been told that my baby is small. How am I going to be monitored?

A1: Counsel this patient about the findings and how you propose to monitor fetal well-being.

Counselling would involve the following points:
- The scan suggests that the baby is small.
- The scan is otherwise normal (normal blood flow measurements and amount of fluid around the baby), and the baby is active.
- It could therefore be that the baby is small and healthy, but it is important to monitor the baby in case the placenta is not working as well as it should and the baby becomes distressed.
- This monitoring will include assessment of the baby's heart beat by external cardiotocography (i.e. a belt attached around her abdomen, which will monitor the heart over a 20-min period). This will be performed every day, but could be done as an outpatient.
- A repeat USS will be performed in 1 week to measure blood flow through the umbilical cord (umbilical arterial Doppler), and in 2 weeks to measure how much the baby has grown and to check growth velocity and again to measure blood flow through the umbilical cord and the amount of fluid around the baby.
- She should monitor the movements of the baby and notify the hospital if there is any change in pattern, particularly a reduction in movements.
- If any concern arises about the condition of the baby while this monitoring is being undertaken (e.g. signs of fetal distress or inadequate growth), early delivery may be required.
- She will be given a course of steroids to help mature the baby's lungs in case early delivery is indicated.

OSCE COUNSELLING CASE 2.2 – I want to have screening for Down's syndrome. What is involved?

A1: Counsel her about screening for Down's syndrome.

As she is only 10 weeks she can be offered first trimester screening. Details of the tests should include the following:
- What is involved (a USS and a venous blood sample).
- When it is performed (between 11 and 14 weeks).
- The USS confirms gestational age and a measurement of the nuchal thickness (NT: skin behind fetal neck) is taken.
- The blood measures two hormones, PAPP-A and free ßhCG and data on levels of these hormones and the NT combined with the mother's age will give a measure of her personal risk of having a Down's syndrome baby. The risk is classified as high (>1:250) or low (<1:250).

General points applicable to ultrasound and biochemical screening:
- How long the results will take to be returned.
- How the patient will receive the results.

- The tests do not diagnose Down's syndrome and, if the patient is in the high-risk category, she will require further investigation (i.e. amniocentesis or chorionic villus sampling – CVS). Both of these tests are associated with excess fetal loss (1 per cent for amniocentesis and 2–3 per cent for CVS).
- If the patient is in the low-risk category, she may still have a baby with Down's syndrome.
- A detailed anomaly scan at 18–20 weeks may identify associated anomalies (e.g. cardiac abnormalities or other 'markers' for Down's syndrome).
- If the patient had a Down's syndrome fetus, would she consider termination of pregnancy? This may affect her decision as to whether to participate in the screening programme but is not a prerequisite.

Box 2.3 Risks of polyhydramnios

- Pre-term labour.
- Pre-term rupture of membranes.
- Cord prolapse.
- Unstable lie.
- Malpresentation.
- Abruptio placentae.
- Postpartum haemorrhage.

REVISION PANEL

- The uterus is usually palpable abdominally at 12–14 weeks' gestation. The uterine fundus reaches the umbilicus at 20 weeks' gestation.
- Dating a pregnancy to confirm gestation with ultrasound is only accurate before 20 weeks' gestation.
- The mainstay of management of intrauterine growth restriction is to deliver a fetus as mature and in as good a condition as possible. A fetus suspected of being growth restricted requires regular assessment of growth and well-being.
- Large for dates pregnancy is not an indication for early delivery or elective caesarean section in its own right i.e. in the absence of additional fetal or maternal concerns.
- Biochemical and ultrasound screening for Down's syndrome only gives a maternal risk. Amniocentesis or CVS is required to confirm a diagnosis.

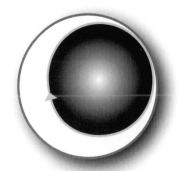

3 Late pregnancy problems

Questions

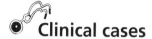

Clinical cases

For each of the case scenarios given, consider the following:

> **Q1**: What is the likely differential diagnosis?
> **Q2**: What issues in the given history support the diagnosis?
> **Q3**: What additional features in the history would you seek to support a particular diagnosis?
> **Q4**: What clinical examination would you perform and why?
> **Q5**: What investigations would be most helpful and why?
> **Q6**: What treatment options are appropriate?

CASE 3.1 – I am 38 weeks pregnant and bleeding vaginally.

A 24-year-old woman attends the midwife at 38 weeks' gestation. She has had two previous uncomplicated deliveries, and she is concerned that over the past few days she has been having a small amount of fresh vaginal bleeding intermittently. She has no abdominal pain and the baby is active.

CASE 3.2 – I have not felt my baby move since yesterday.

A 30-year-old parous woman at 36 weeks' gestation has not felt any fetal movements on the day when she presents to the doctor. Fetal movements had been becoming less frequent over the last few days, but she had not been recording them. She previously had two normal deliveries at term of babies of normal weight. In this pregnancy her scans showed a singleton fetus consistent with menstrual dates at 12 weeks and with no fetal anomaly at 20 weeks. Her screening for Down's syndrome was reported as low risk. She has been managed as a low-risk patient, because her pregnancy has progressed without any problems.

CASE 3.3 – I am 32 weeks' pregnant and am having abdominal pain and contractions.

A 25-year-old nulliparous woman at 32 weeks' gestation presents with abdominal pain associated with uterine contractions. Fetal movements are satisfactory. Her booking ultrasound scan (USS) showed singleton pregnancy consistent with menstrual dates and her anomaly scan at 20 weeks' gestation was normal. Her screening for Down's syndrome was reported as low risk. She had been a smoker but stopped in mid-trimester. She had an appendectomy as a child. She was assessed to be a low-risk pregnancy at booking.

⁇ OSCE counselling cases

OSCE COUNSELLING CASE 3.1 – **I have experienced bleeding in pregnancy. How will I be managed?**

An 18-year-old woman has had one episode of unprovoked fresh vaginal bleeding at 28 weeks' gestation. A USS shows a normally growing fetus with a placenta sited in the lower segment as a minor (grade I) placenta praevia. The patient has no abdominal tenderness. Her cardiotocograph (CTG) is normal, her haemoglobin 12.0 g/dL and her blood group rhesus negative. She has been in the hospital for a few days and the bleeding has not recurred.

Q1: What information is required for counselling this patient about how she will be managed during the rest of her pregnancy?

OSCE COUNSELLING CASE 3.2 – **How should I record fetal movements?**

A 29-year-old woman presents with reduced fetal movements at 35 weeks' gestation. Investigations show a normal CTG.

Q1: What information is required for counselling this patient about monitoring her fetal movements over the next few weeks?

Answers

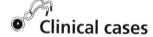

Clinical cases

CASE 3.1 – I am 38 weeks pregnant and bleeding vaginally.

A1: What is the likely differential diagnosis?
- Placenta praevia (Fig. 3.1).
- Placental abruption.
- Cervical lesion (e.g. erosion, polyp, cancer).

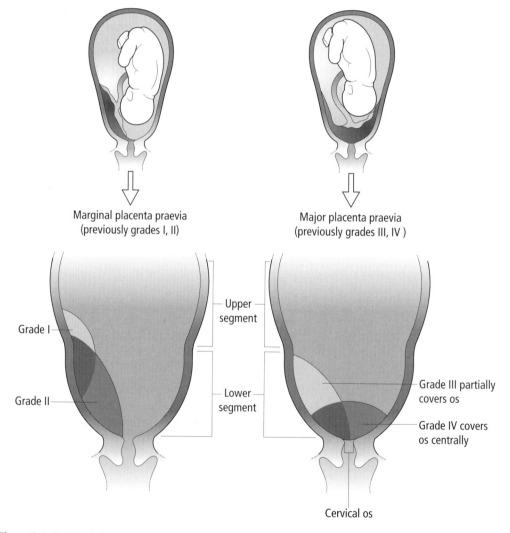

Figure 3.1 Grades of placenta praevia.

A2: What issues in the given history support the diagnosis?

The history of painless small bleeds supports the diagnosis of placenta praevia.

A3: What additional features in the history would you seek to support a particular diagnosis?

The patient's smear history should be obtained. The reports of any previous USSs in this pregnancy should be checked in order to identify the location of the placenta.

A4: What clinical examination would you perform and why?

The pulse and blood pressure should be recorded.
- Examination would include abdominal palpation, with a soft non-tender uterus, high presenting part and an abnormal lie supporting a diagnosis of placenta praevia, and a tense tender uterus supporting a diagnosis of placental abruption.
- The fetal heart should be auscultated to exclude fetal distress, which is more commonly associated with placental abruption.
- If it is confirmed that the placenta is not low (by USS), a speculum examination to visualize the cervix and look for local causes, e.g. erosion/cancer would be indicated. Under no circumstances should a digital examination be performed, because torrential bleeding can be provoked if a placenta praevia has falsely been excluded as a cause.

A5: What investigations would be most helpful and why?

• **FBC**	✓	To identify the presence of anaemia.
• **Blood group and cross-match/ Kleihauer test if rhesus negative**	✓	In case bleeding increases and a transfusion is required. The patient should be given anti-D if her blood group is rhesus negative to prevent isoimmunization.
• **USS**	✓	To localize the placenta and determine whether it is low lying, as well as to assess fetal growth and well-being.
• **CTG**	✓	To identify fetal compromise.

A6: What treatment options are appropriate?

Management would be to admit the patient to an obstetric unit. At term gestation with a history of antepartum haemorrhage, delivery is indicated to ensure the safe delivery of a mature fetus.
- Caesarean section should be performed in cases of major placenta praevia.
- Consider examination without anaesthesia and artificial rupture of membranes in cases with minor degrees of placenta praevia. This procedure should be performed in an operating theatre with a senior anaesthetist present and ready to administer a general anaesthetic to expedite delivery if bleeding is provoked on vaginal examination. In addition, cross-matched blood should be available in the operating theatre and scrub nurses should be ready to perform an immediate caesarean section (i.e. scrubbed with instrument tray open).

- If a diagnosis of placental abruption is suspected (based on the absence of a low lying placenta on scan, normal appearance of the cervix on speculum examination) and there is no evidence of fetal compromise, an artificial rupture of the membranes should be performed and an oxytocin (Syntocinon) infusion commenced with continuous monitoring of the fetal heart because of the increased risk of fetal hypoxia. If fetal compromise is suspected a caesarean section should be performed.

Box 3.1 Risks of antepartum haemorrhage

- Haemorrhage and shock with placenta praevia and placental abruption.
- Renal failure due to hypovolaemic shock.
- Disseminated intravascular coagulation (DIC) in placental abruption or in cases of major blood loss in placenta praevia.
- Fetal hypoxia.
- Intrauterine death.

CASE 3.2 – I have not felt my baby move since yesterday.

A1: What is the likely differential diagnosis?

- Prolonged periods of fetal sleep without any compromise.
- Fetal compromise.
- Fetal death.

A2: What issues in the given history support the diagnosis?

In most cases with the given history, there is no particular obstetric problem. In this case, the pregnancy had been uncomplicated. Reduced movements had been reported over several days, which would warrant further investigation in order to exclude fetal compromise or death.

A3: What additional features in the history would you seek to support a particular diagnosis?

The history should explore whether there are any reasons (e.g. hypertension, diabetes, fetal growth retardation and haemorrhage) for concern about fetal compromise.

A4: What clinical examination would you perform and why?

A general examination, including pulse, temperature (sepsis associated with intrauterine fetal death) and blood pressure (associated pre-eclampsia), is required. The abdomen should be examined to determine the symphysiofundal height, and clinical assessment of liquor volume should be made (fetal compromise is associated with growth restriction and reduced liquor volume). Try to stimulate fetal movements by gently moving the fetus around at the time of abdominal palpation. Listen to the fetal heart to exclude fetal death. If no fetal heart is heard a USS is required.

A5: What investigations would be most helpful and why?

- **Urinalysis** ☑ To exclude proteinuria to detect pre-eclampsia.

- **CTG** ☑ To assess fetal well-being, looking for variability, accelerations and a lack of decelerations.

- **USS** ± Required only if there is concern about fetal growth or well-being, to (1) check fetal heart rate and (2) assess fetal well-being by assessing liquor volume, fetal movements (which may not be perceived by the patient), fetal tone, fetal respiration and umbilical Doppler (absent or reversed diastolic flow) biophysical profile.

A6: What treatment options are appropriate?

- Confirm fetal well-being, and, if this is satisfactory, the patient can be discharged home with advice to record daily fetal movements (using a kick chart). If there are fewer than 10 movements over a 12-h period, the patient will need to return for a CTG.
- If there is fetal growth restriction, investigations will be performed to identify fetal compromise. As the pregnancy is approaching term, delivery may be contemplated.
- If fetal death is confirmed, medical induction of pregnancy should be conducted using antiprogestogens and prostaglandins together with appropriate investigations (fetal postmortem examination, chromosome analysis of fetus and parents, anticardiolipin antibodies, lupus and infection screen) and bereavement counselling.

CASE 3.3 – I am 32 weeks' pregnant and am having abdominal pain and contractions.

A1: What is the likely differential diagnosis?

- Obstetric causes:
  - pre-term labour;
  - chorioamnionitis;
  - concealed abruptio placentae;
  - fibroid degeneration (usually at mid-trimester).
- Non-obstetric causes:
  - urinary tract infection, pyelonephritis (can precipitate preterm labour);
  - irritable bowel syndrome, constipation;
  - ovarian cyst (haemorrhage, torsion).

A2: What issues in the given history support the diagnosis?

The history seems to suggest preterm labour. There are many causes of preterm labour including infection, placental abruption, idiopathic and multiple pregnancy. Smoking is a risk factor for abruptio placentae, which may lead to preterm labour.

A3: What additional features in the history would you seek to support a particular diagnosis?

The history should first establish whether the uterine activity is regular or irregular and whether or not it is painful. Irregular uterine action is not usually associated with labour and is likely to be Braxton Hicks contractions, particularly if not associated with pain. Regular, painful contractions that progressively become longer, more painful and more frequent are typically labour pains. Lack of pain-free intervals would suggest abruptio placentae. Vaginal bleeding is often (but not always, as in concealed abruption) associated with abruptio placentae. A history of ruptured membranes supports the diagnosis of chorioamnionitis. A history of urinary symptoms (dysuria, loin pain, etc.) and bowel symptoms (vomiting, diarrhoea, etc.) might suggest a non-obstetric cause of the problem. However, these conditions can sometimes precipitate preterm labour. Ureteric colic can mimic labour pains. A history of fibroids on scan might suggest red degeneration, especially if the pain is localized.

A4: What clinical examination would you perform and why?

A general examination, including pulse, temperature and blood pressure, is required. The abdomen should be examined to determine uterine irritability and contractility, and the duration of contractions should be determined and the loins examined for tenderness. Symphysiofundal height should be measured and liquor volume should be clinically assessed. Fetal presentation and lie should be examined (this influences the mode of delivery). Uterine tenderness may be associated with abruptio placentae or chorioamnionitis. Listen to the fetal heart because abruption (heart rate decelerations) or chorioamnionitis (tachycardia) is associated with fetal compromise. Vaginal examination should be performed under aseptic conditions to establish the diagnosis of labour. Labour is more likely if the cervical os is dilating, the cervix is effaced (short in length) and the membranes have ruptured.

A5: What investigations would be most helpful and why?

● **FBC**	☑	For anaemia and/or neutrophilia with the latter being an indication of infection.
● **CRP**	☑	To exclude infection.
● **Urinalysis and culture**	☑	To exclude urinary tract infection.
● **CTG**	☑	To assess fetal well-being. Recording of contractions on antenatal CTG provides information only about their frequency, and not about their intensity.
● **USS**	☑	USS to check fetal well-being and assess liquor volume (which may be reduced if membranes are ruptured).
● **Coagulation screen**	☑	If abruptio placentae is suspected.
● **Blood group and cross-match**	☑	If abruptio placentae is suspected.
● **Kleihauer test**	±	If abruptio placentae is suspected and patient is rhesus negative.
● **HVS**	☑	For infection, e.g. group B streptococcus, particularly if there is vaginal discharge or ruptured membranes.

A6: What treatment options are appropriate?

● In preterm labour, management aims to suppress uterine activity and prolong pregnancy (if the maternal and fetal conditions allow this) in order to administer steroids, which reduce the incidence and severity of respiratory distress syndrome. This can be achieved by tocolysis using the oxytocin receptor antagonist atosiban, the ß-agonist ritodrine, the calcium antagonist nifedipine or the prostaglandin synthase inhibitor indometacin. The most commonly used agent is atosiban. Indometacin and ritodrine have adverse side effect profiles. Indometacin can result in transient impairment of fetal renal function and premature closure of the ductus arteriosus. Ritodrine can cause side effects in the mother, including tachycardia, pulmonary oedema and arrhythmias. Nifedipine is not licensed for this use. Tocolytics should be given for 24–48h only to allow the administration of steroids.

- If abruptio placentae is suspected, it should be managed according to maternal and fetal well-being. If there is no maternal shock or concern regarding fetal well-being, a conservative approach can be adopted. Administer steroids, but do not attempt to suppress labour. If immediate delivery is indicated, decide on the mode of delivery, bearing in mind maternal and fetal condition, progress of labour, and fetal presentation and lie.
- If there is suspected infection, give antibiotics and augment labour if there is clinical evidence of chorioamnionitis.
- *In utero* transfer will be required if there are no neonatal intensive care facilities on site.

👥 OSCE counselling cases

OSCE COUNSELLING CASE 3.1 – **I have experienced bleeding in pregnancy. How will I be managed?**

A1: What information is required for counselling this patient about how she will be managed during the rest of her pregnancy?

- This patient has minor placenta praevia (grades I and II), which is likely to be the cause of her antepartum haemorrhage. Steroids should be administered for fetal lung maturity as there is a risk of need for preterm delivery. Tocolysis is generally contraindicated in antepartum haemorrhage. There is no need for long-term hospitalization, which would be necessary only for major placenta praevia (grades III and IV).
- There is no cause for concern because the bleeding has stopped. However, there is a risk of recurrence and potential need for preterm delivery.
- If there is no further bleeding, placental site and fetal growth should be checked by USS at 34 weeks' gestation.
- If there is further bleeding after the patient has been discharged home, she should return to hospital immediately.
- If the placenta is no longer low lying at the 34-week scan, the remainder of the pregnancy will be treated as low risk.
- If the placenta remains low lying at 34 weeks, serial 2-weekly scans should be performed for placental site. If subsequent scans show the placenta not to be low lying, the remainder of the pregnancy will be treated as low risk.
- If the placenta remains low lying at term the approach to delivery needs to be considered (see Case 3.1).
- Advise against intercourse.
- A Kleihauer test should be performed and an appropriate dose of anti-D given.

OSCE COUNSELLING CASE 3.2 – **How should I record fetal movements?**

A1: What information is required for counselling this patient about monitoring her fetal movements over the next few weeks?

- A kick chart is the established method for monitoring fetal movement.
- This chart reassures the patient that all is well, and allows her to identify potential problems in an objective way.
- Specific instructions on how to use the chart include the following:
  - begin at 09:00;
  - count every separate movement and record it on the chart with a tick;
  - if the baby has not moved at least 10 times by 18:00, the patient should attend the labour suite;
  - in the labour suite the patient will undergo cardiotocography and other investigations if required;
  - further management will depend on the findings of these tests, and they might warrant expediting delivery (see Case 3.2).
- Smoking, dehydration and poor food intake can reduce fetal movements.
- Warn the patient that, with increasing gestation, the time taken to detect the full 10 movements will become longer. This is normal as long as the 10 movements occur before 18:00.

REVISION PANEL

- In cases of antepartum haemorrhage a speculum examination should not be undertaken until a placenta praevia has been excluded on ultrasound scan.
- Anti-D should be administered to unsensitised Rhesus negative women with antepartum haemorrhage to prevent Rhesus isoimmunisation.
- In cases of placental abruption concealed haemorrhage can be underestimated resulting in inadequate resuscitation and hence increased risk of complications of hypovolaemia.
- In cases of threatened pre-term labour maternal steroids should be administered to reduce the risk and severity of respiratory distress syndrome in the baby if delivery ensues.

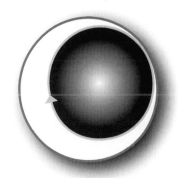

4 Labour

Questions

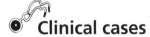

Clinical cases

For each of the case scenarios given, consider the following:

Q1: What is the likely differential diagnosis?
Q2: What issues in the given history support the diagnosis?
Q3: What additional features in the history would you seek to support a particular diagnosis?
Q4: What clinical examination would you perform and why?
Q5: What investigations would be most helpful and why?
Q6: What treatment options are appropriate?

CASE 4.1 – **My baby is due and I am having contractions.**

A 22-year-old primigravida with a singleton pregnancy at term has had an uncomplicated pregnancy. She starts to have regular uterine contractions and telephones the labour suite. On the advice of a midwife, she makes her way to the hospital.

CASE 4.2 – **I am in labour and the midwife says my baby is getting tired.**

A 20-year-old, unemployed, single mother has had labour induced at 38 weeks' gestation because the baby was considered to be growth restricted. This is her first pregnancy and she smokes 20 cigarettes per day. The cervix is dilated 4 cm, and the midwife is concerned about the cardiotocograph (CTG) (Fig. 4.1).

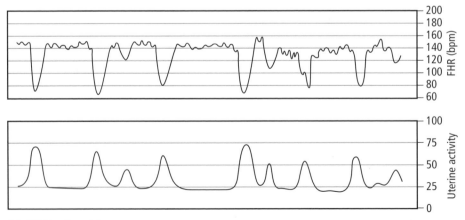

Figure 4.1 CTG for Case 4.2.

CASE 4.3 – The midwife says my labour is not progressing.

A 26-year-old primigravida at term is in spontaneous labour. Her height is 172 cm. Her pregnancy has been uncomplicated. She has a singleton pregnancy with a cephalic presentation and the vertex is engaged. She has not required analgesia. Her partogram is shown in Fig. 4.2.

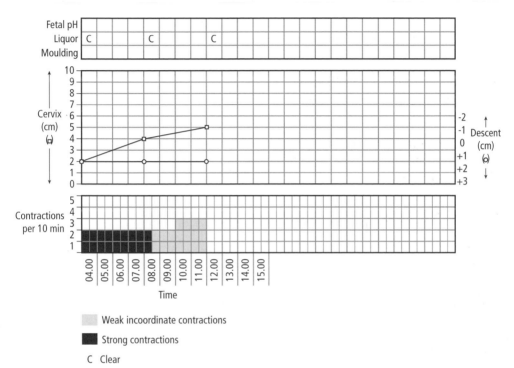

Figure 4.2 Partogram for Case 4.3.

CASE 4.4 – The midwife says my labour is not progressing.

A 26-year-old primigravida at term is in spontaneous labour. She has a singleton pregnancy with a longitudinal lie and a cephalic presentation. Her previous pregnancy ended at 34 weeks with a spontaneous vaginal delivery of a 2.0 kg baby. Her height is 150 cm. Her pregnancy has been uncomplicated, but the midwife has often said that 'the baby feels big'. She has been in labour all day and her partogram is shown in Fig. 4.3. She has been given oxytocin (Syntocinon) for the last 4 h.

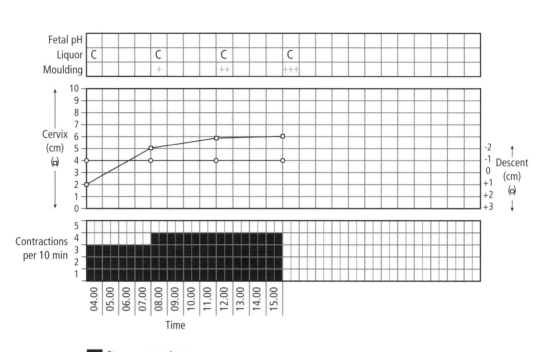

Figure 4.3 Partogram for Case 4.4.

ii OSCE counselling cases

OSCE COUNSELLING CASE 4.1 – **What pain relief should I have in labour?**

A primigravida, who is attending her first antenatal clinic, wishes to know more about the pain relief that will be available to her during labour.

Q1: What are the options for pain relief during labour?

OSCE COUNSELLING CASE 4.2 – **I have passed my due date and I am not in labour yet.**

A primigravida attends her antenatal clinic at 42 weeks. The pregnancy was dated by ultrasound scan (USS) in the second trimester and she has had a normal antenatal course. The fetus is well grown and lying longitudinally with cephalic presentation. The mother wishes to have labour induced. Apart from some irregular uterine contractions, she has not gone into labour spontaneously.

Q1: What information will be required for counselling her about induction of labour for post-term pregnancy?

🔑 Key concepts

In order to work through the core clinical cases in this chapter, you will need to understand the following key concepts.

STAGES OF LABOUR
- First stage: from the onset of regular painful contractions until full dilatation of the cervix.
- Second stage: from full dilatation of the cervix until delivery of the baby.
- Third stage: from delivery of the baby until delivery of the placenta.

FETAL LIE
The relationship of the long axis of the fetus with that of the mother (e.g. longitudinal/transverse).

PRESENTATION
The part of the fetus that occupies the lower segment of the uterus (e.g. cephalic when the head occupies the lower segment).

PRESENTING PART
The lowest part of the fetus that is palpable on vaginal examination.

POSITION
The position of the fetal presenting part in the maternal pelvis in relation to the 'denominator': the occiput in a vertex presentation and the sacrum in a breech presentation (e.g. occipitoanterior, sacroposterior).

VERTEX
The area of the fetal skull that is bordered by the anterior fontanelle, the posterior fontanelle and the parietal eminences.

ENGAGEMENT
The state when the widest diameter of the fetal presenting part enters the maternal pelvis.

STATION
Descent of the presenting part measured in centimetres above or below the level of the ischial spines.

ATTITUDE
The degree of flexion of the fetal head (e.g. vertex, brow or face).

MOULDING
The reduction in the diameters of the fetal head caused by the coming together, or overlapping, of the sutures in the fetal skull as the head is compressed by the maternal pelvis.

CAPUT
Localized swelling of the fetal scalp secondary to pressure during labour.

POSTPARTUM HAEMORRHAGE
- Primary: the loss of >500 mL of blood within 24 h of delivery.
- Secondary: the loss of >500 mL of blood after 24 h and within 6 weeks of delivery.

CERVICAL EFFACEMENT

The length of cervix that shortens to indicate that labour has started. In primiparous women, the cervix is tubular and gets 'drawn up' into the lower segment until it is flat.

BISHOP SCORE

A measure of the 'favourability' of the cervix for induction of labour (Table 4.1). The lower the score, the more unfavourable the cervix.

Table 4.1 Bishop score

Points	0	1	2	3	Score
Dilatation (cm)	0	1–2	3–4	5–6	
Cervical canal length (cm)	2	1–2	0.5–1	<0.5	
Station	–3	–2	–1/0	+1/+2	
Consistency	Firm	Medium	Soft		
Position	Posterior	Mid	Anterior		
					Total

Answers

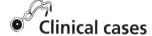

Clinical cases

CASE 4.1 – **My baby is due and I am having contractions.**

A1: What is the likely differential diagnosis?
- Labour.
- Braxton Hicks contractions.
- 'False labour'.

A2: What issues in the given history support the diagnosis?
Regular uterine contractions at term usually indicate the start of spontaneous labour.

A3: What additional features in the history would you seek to support a particular diagnosis?
Increasing regularity and duration of contractions would support a diagnosis of the onset of spontaneous labour. A 'show' (mucus plug from the cervix) and/or rupture of the membranes may accompany the onset of labour. A brief history of the current pregnancy should be taken.

A4: What clinical examination would you perform and why?
A general assessment of maternal condition is made, including measurement of pulse, blood pressure and temperature. Abdominal palpation is performed to feel for uterine contractions, confirm the lie and presentation, check for engagement of the presenting part and listen to the fetal heart. A vaginal examination is performed to check for cervical effacement and dilatation, station and position of the presenting part, and the colour of any liquor draining. Labour would be confirmed if regular uterine contractions were present in association with an effacing and dilating cervix and descent of the presenting part.

A5: What investigations would be most helpful and why?
- **Urinalysis** ☑ Proteinuria is evidence of pre-eclampsia if associated with raised blood pressure and can arise for the first time in labour. Ketonuria is evidence of dehydration.

A6: What treatment options are appropriate?
- Maternal well-being should be assessed by regular measurement of the patient's temperature, pulse and blood pressure, which should all be recorded on a partogram. Dehydration should be avoided, with the patient being encouraged to drink water. As a result of the delayed gastric emptying time and the risk of aspiration, food should be avoided during labour. The mother should be encouraged to micturate frequently in labour to enable measurement of urine output and to avoid urinary retention. On each occasion the urine can also be tested for protein and ketones.

- Fetal well-being should be assessed by observing the colour of the liquor. The presence of meconium might indicate fetal hypoxia. The fetal heart should be auscultated every 15 min during and for 1 min after a contraction. If an abnormality is detected, or if another indication arises (e.g. epidural analgesia is used), continuous fetal heart rate monitoring should be commenced.
- Progress of labour should be assessed by performing regular (4-hourly) vaginal examinations. The dilatation of the cervix is estimated in centimetres, the descent of the head is measured by its relationship to the ischial spines as centimetres above or below an imaginary line drawn between the spines, and these measurements are recorded on a partogram (see Figs. 4.2 and 4.3).
- Adequate pain relief should be provided. Transcutaneous electrical nerve stimulation (TENS), Entonox, opiates (e.g. pethidine, diamorphine) and an epidural block are commonly used options. The choice will depend on maternal preference in association with factors such as the stage of labour, the availability of an anaesthetist if an epidural is chosen and other obstetric factors (e.g. hypertension, in which case an epidural may be more appropriate).

CASE 4.2 – **I am in labour and the midwife says my baby is getting tired.**

A1: What is the likely differential diagnosis?

Suspected fetal distress in labour.

A2: What issues in the given history support the diagnosis?

Fetal growth restriction is a risk factor for fetal hypoxia. The CTG in this case is abnormal, with reduced beat-to-beat variation, no accelerations and variable decelerations.

A3: What additional features in the history would you seek to support a particular diagnosis?

Additional risk factors for intrauterine growth restriction in which hypoxia is more common include smoking, elevated blood pressure, antepartum haemorrhage and chronic maternal disease (e.g. renal disease). Reduced fetal movements may have been noted before the induction of labour. Meconium-stained liquor during labour may be associated with fetal hypoxia.

Box 4.1 Meconium staining of liquor

- Meconium staining is present in 15 per cent of all deliveries at term and in 40 per cent of deliveries post-term.
- Meconium staining of liquor is associated with, but not always a sign of, fetal hypoxia.
- Gross meconium staining is likely to be significant and, together with CTG abnormalities, should never be ignored.
- Meconium aspiration by the baby may cause pneumonitis, which can be fatal. Aspirating the upper airway at the time of delivery to clear meconium can reduce the risk of this occurring.

A4: What clinical examination would you perform and why?

Examination would include abdominal palpation, where the fetal size as assessed by the symphysiofundal measurement may be less than expected for gestational age. This finding would support fetal growth restriction with fetal hypoxia.

A5: What investigations would be most helpful and why?

● **Fetal blood sampling**   ☑   The reduced beat-to-beat variation and variable decelerations would give cause for concern (Box 4.2).

Box 4.2 What should be done when irregularities of the CTG occur?

● A significant proportion of babies who are thought to have 'fetal distress' as determined by abnormalities on the CTG and who are subsequently delivered by forceps or caesarean section are not hypoxic. A normal CTG, however, is very reassuring and indicates good fetal well-being.
● In cases where CTG monitoring shows signs that raise the possibility of fetal hypoxia (e.g. tachycardia, decelerations), this should be confirmed by fetal scalp blood sampling to measure fetal pH and base excess.

A6: What treatment options are appropriate?

Management would be according to the analysis of fetal blood sampling (Box 4.3).

Box 4.3 Obstetric management after fetal blood sample

pH <7.20

Deliver the baby by forceps/ventouse if the cervix is fully dilated and the fetal head is engaged, or by caesarean section if this is not the case.

pH >7.20 but <7.25

Repeat fetal blood sampling after 30 min, unless there is a deterioration in CTG before this time.

pH >7.25

Normal result: repeat fetal blood sampling if CTG deteriorates.

CASE 4.3 – **The midwife says my labour is not progressing.**

A1: What is the likely differential diagnosis?

Failure to progress in labour may result from:
● Inadequate uterine activity.
● Absolute or relative cephalopelvic disproportion, i.e. baby too big/pelvis too small or fetal head in malposition.

A2: What issues in the given history support the diagnosis?

Her height (no evidence of short stature) and the fact that the vertex is engaged do not support cephalopelvic disproportion. The lack of requirement for analgesia would support inadequate uterine contractions.

A3: What additional features in the history would you seek to support a particular diagnosis?

The frequency and duration of contractions should be recorded. Risk factors for cephalopelvic disproportion (e.g. macrosomia, diabetes) should be sought.

A4: What clinical examination would you perform and why?

Examination would include an abdominal palpation to assess the clinical size of the baby, to assess the amount of head that is palpable in order to determine whether the head is engaged, and also to assess the frequency and strength of uterine contractions. Four-hourly vaginal examinations should be performed to assess the progress of labour, and the findings should be plotted on a partogram (as shown in Fig. 4.2). Assessment of fetal position should be made as a malposition (e.g. persistent occipitoposterior) would create a relative cephalopelvic disproportion because of the increased diameters presented. An assessment of the presence and degree of moulding (overlapping skull bones) and caput (scalp oedema) is required and would support cephalopelvic disproportion, if present. An assessment of liquor colour should be made, with the presence of meconium indicating the possibility of fetal hypoxia. Maternal well-being (pulse, blood pressure, temperature, urine output) should be assessed and adequate analgesia provided.

A5: What investigations would be most helpful and why?

• **CTG**	✓	To look for evidence of associated fetal distress.
• **FBC**	✓	To check for anaemia in case caesarean section is required.
• **Group and save blood**	✓	In case caesarean section is required and a transfusion becomes necessary as a result.

A6: What treatment options are appropriate?

In this case the diagnosis is incoordinate/infrequent uterine contractions. There is no caput or moulding to suggest cephalopelvic disproportion. Commence oxytocin (Syntocinon) and reassess in 4h if there is still no concern about fetal condition. Oxytocin makes the contractions more regular, stronger and more frequent, resulting in effective uterine contractions that will lead to cervical dilatation and fetal head descent.

CASE 4.4 – **The midwife says my labour is not progressing.**

A1: What is the likely differential diagnosis?

Failure to progress in labour may result from:
- Cephalopelvic disproportion.
- Poor uterine contractility.

A2: What issues in the given history support the diagnosis?

Her height (short stature) and the fact that her baby is clinically large (macrosomic) point towards cephalopelvic disproportion. Her uterine contractions are adequate as recorded on the partogram.

A3: What additional features in the history would you seek to support a particular diagnosis?

Consider predisposing factors for macrosomia (e.g. gestational diabetes).

A4: What clinical examination would you perform and why?

Examination would include an abdominal palpation to assess the clinical size of the baby and to assess the amount of fetal head that is palpable in order to determine whether the head is engaged. The frequency and strength of uterine contractions also need to be assessed. Four-hourly vaginal examinations would be performed to assess the progress of labour, and the findings should be plotted on a partogram. At vaginal examination, assessment of the position of the vertex would be required as a malposition (e.g. persistent occipitoposterior) could create a relative cephalopelvic disproportion because of the increased fetal diameters presented to the maternal pelvis. An assessment should be made of the degree of moulding (overlapping skull bones) and caput (scalp oedema), the presence of which would support cephalopelvic disproportion. The colour of the liquor should be noted, with the presence of meconium indicating the possibility of fetal hypoxia. Assessment should also be made of maternal well-being and adequate pain relief should be provided.

A5: What investigations would be most helpful and why?

● **CTG**	✓	To look for evidence of associated fetal distress.
● **FBC**	✓	To check for anaemia in case caesarean section is required.
● **Group and save blood**	✓	In case caesarean section is required and a transfusion becomes necessary as a result.

A6: What treatment options are appropriate?

In this case the diagnosis is cephalopelvic disproportion. Caesarean section under spinal or epidural anaesthesia is required because, according to the partogram, the cervix has not dilated for 4 h, the fetal head has not descended in the maternal pelvis and labour has not progressed despite 4 h of uterine stimulation with oxytocin.

ii OSCE counselling cases

OSCE COUNSELLING CASE 4.1 – **What pain relief should I have in labour?**

A1: What are the options for pain relief during labour?

- Antenatal preparation and a calm labour environment are important. The presence of a partner or birth attendant who can rub and/or massage the woman's back and provide reassurance and support can help during labour. Attendance at parent-craft classes will help the woman to prepare for labour.
- Choices of analgesia in labour include the following:
    - transcutaneous electrical nerve stimulation can be of benefit in early labour;
    - Entonox inhalation has a rapid onset with mild analgesic effects. It is most effective in early labour. It is best to start inhaling before the onset of a contraction and to continue until the end of the contraction. It can cause light-headedness and nausea;
    - opiates such as pethidine and diamorphine can be given as an intramuscular injection every 4–6 h. Pethidine has central sedative effects rather than providing effective analgesia. Patients can therefore become confused and feel 'out of control'. It also causes nausea, so there is often a need for antiemetics. It can cause a sleep pattern in the fetus, so the fetal heart rate may show some abnormality. At birth, respiratory depression can also occur in the neonate. Diamorphine given in a similar fashion has a stronger analgesic effect;
    - epidural analgesia with or without opiates is a very effective form of analgesia that can be either given intermittently or infused continuously via a pump. It completely blocks sensation (except pressure) and induces partial motor blockade, making the legs feel heavy and 'dead', so mobility is restricted. It is useful if surgical delivery is required.
- Maternal choice and input in decision making is important. Other factors, e.g. parity, stage of labour, or other complications, such as hypertension, should be taken into account as they will influence the best option for pain relief.

OSCE COUNSELLING CASE 4.2 – **I have passed my due date and I am not in labour yet.**

A1: What information will be required for counselling her about induction of labour for post-term pregnancy?

- Post-term pregnancy occurs in about 10 per cent of pregnant women.
- One approach to management of this condition is to monitor fetal well-being while awaiting spontaneous labour, but it is reasonable to induce labour as an alternative. It is recommended that induction of labour should be offered at term +7–14 days, in the interest of the fetus, with perinatal deaths being more common after this period.
- On admission to hospital, fetal well-being should be assessed with a CTG.
- The state of the cervix will be examined in order to determine its length, dilatation, consistency and position (a score can be calculated in combination with the station of the fetal head – see Table 4.1 for Bishop score). If the cervix is favourable for induction (Bishop score >6), the fetal membranes can be ruptured artificially (artificial rupture of membranes or ARM), which would result in a significant proportion of women going into labour a short time afterwards.

- If the cervix is not favourable for induction (Bishop score <6), prostaglandin is administered in the form of vaginal pessaries. The prostaglandin usually softens and effaces the cervix. Sometimes it can initiate labour, but its main role in this situation is to ripen the cervix before ARM.
- If ARM does not initiate labour, the latter may be induced or augmented with oxytocin (Syntocinon) infusion.
- If induction of labour fails completely, a caesarean delivery may be performed.
- Labour after successful induction is managed in the usual manner with regard to pain relief, assessment of maternal well-being, and progress of labour. However, continuous fetal heart rate monitoring should be performed.

Box 4.4 Post-dates pregnancy

- Perinatal mortality increases by twofold after 42 weeks.
- The caesarean section rate increases by twofold after 42 weeks.
- Meconium staining occurs in 40 per cent of pregnancies beyond 42 weeks.
- Caesarean section rates increase in association with induction of labour in post-dates pregnancy, together with an unripe cervix.

REVISION PANEL

- The Bishop score is a measure of the 'favourability' of the cervix for induction of labour. The lower the score, the more unfavourable the cervix. An unfavourable cervix should be primed with prostaglandins if there is no contraindication prior to attempt at induction of labour.
- The partogram is a tool to record the progress of labour and assist in decision-making regarding the management of labour. It should be completed prospectively for all labours.
- Meconium staining is present in 15 per cent of all deliveries at term and in 40 per cent of deliveries post-term. It is associated with but not diagnostic of hypoxia.
- Failure to progress in labour is associated with problems with one or more of the three 'P's – powers (contractions, i.e. inadequate), passenger (baby, i.e. too large or malposition), passages (pelvis, i.e. too small).
- Post-term pregnancy occurs in about 10 per cent of pregnant women. Perinatal mortality increases by twofold after 42 weeks.

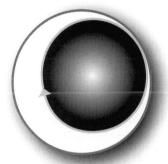

5 Medical disorders of pregnancy

Questions

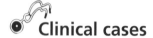

Clinical cases

For each of the case scenarios given, consider the following:

Q1: What is the likely differential diagnosis?
Q2: What issues in the given history support the diagnosis?
Q3: What additional features in the history would you seek to support a particular diagnosis?
Q4: What clinical examination would you perform and why?
Q5: What investigations would be most helpful and why?
Q6: What treatment options are appropriate?

CASE 5.1 – I am pregnant and the midwife says my blood pressure is high.

A 20-year-old primigravida attends the antenatal clinic at 34 weeks' gestation and is noted to have a blood pressure of 150/95 mmHg. Urinalysis is negative. Her blood pressure (BP) had previously been recorded in the range 130–150 to 70–80 mmHg in the mid-trimester. Her booking BP was 120/70 mmHg. The fetus was clinically an appropriate size for dates. Three days later, her blood pressure is 160/100 mmHg and she has developed '++' proteinuria on dipstick testing.

CASE 5.2 – I am 28 weeks pregnant and have sugar in my urine.

A 38-year-old woman with two previous normal deliveries is at 28 weeks' gestation. Her weight is 102 kg. Her pregnancy has been progressing well. She attends the antenatal clinic for a routine visit and on urinalysis is noted to have '+++' glucose in her urine.

CASE 5.3 – I am pregnant and also anaemic.

A 28-year-old vegetarian woman attended the antenatal booking clinic at 12 weeks' gestation. Her five children are aged between 6 months and 8 years. Her haemoglobin level was noted to be 8.5 g/dL.

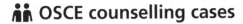 OSCE counselling cases

OSCE COUNSELLING CASE 5.1 – **I have diabetes and want to become pregnant.**

A 23-year-old woman with type 1 diabetes is taking the combined oral contraceptive (COC) pill. She wants to come off the pill to try for a pregnancy.

Q1: What pre-pregnancy counselling would you provide for this woman?

OSCE COUNSELLING CASE 5.2 – **I have epilepsy and I want to become pregnant.**

A 26-year-old woman who has epilepsy controlled by treatment is planning to get married. She is concerned about pregnancy and her epileptic medication. She has been seizure-free for 6 years on two antiepileptic drugs. She has not recently been reviewed by a neurologist.

Q1: What pre-pregnancy care and counselling would you give this woman?

Answers

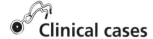

Clinical cases

CASE 5.1 – I am pregnant and the midwife says my blood pressure is high.

A1: What is the likely differential diagnosis?

- Pre-eclampsia (pregnancy-induced proteinuric hypertension).
- Essential hypertension.
- Hypertension secondary to another medical condition (e.g. renal disease or diabetes).

A2: What issues in the given history support the diagnosis?

Pre-eclampsia: based on the fact that the woman's blood pressure is >140/90 mmHg with significant proteinuria. She is a primigravida and pre-eclampsia is more common among such women. Her booking BP was normal.

A3: What additional features in the history would you seek to support a particular diagnosis?

- Any related symptoms (e.g. headache, visual disturbances, epigastric pain) that indicate worsening disease.
- Past history of medical disorders that might cause hypertension (e.g. renal disease or diabetes).
- Previous blood pressure recording to rule out pre-existing essential hypertension, e.g. at her GP, if taking the oral contraceptive.

A4: What clinical examination would you perform and why?

Examination would include fundoscopy to identify hypertensive retinopathy. The reflexes should be examined to identify hyperreflexia and ankle clonus, which would indicate severe pre-eclampsia or impending eclampsia. An abdominal examination may identify right hypochondrial or epigastric tenderness. Ankles and sacral area can be examined for dependent oedema.

A5: What investigations would be most helpful and why?

● **U&Es**	☑	To identify renal compromise.
● **Urate**	☑	Rising plasma urate levels indicate worsening disease.
● **FBC**	☑	A fall in platelet count indicates worsening disease.
● **LFT**	±	If clinically indicated (i.e. worsening blood pressure or increased proteinuria), investigation may include LFTs to identify the presence of HELLP (haemolysis, elevated liver enzymes and low platelets) syndrome, an indication of worsening disease and imminent eclampsia.

- **Urinalysis** ☑ Twice daily urinalysis for proteinuria; 24-h urinary protein may also be measured. Levels of >300 mg/24 h are abnormal.

- **USS** ☑ To assess growth and well-being. Hypertensive disorders of pregnancy are associated with intrauterine restricted growth (IUGR).

- **CTG** ☑ To assess fetal well-being.

A6: What treatment options are appropriate?

Pre-eclampsia is usually a progressive condition. Treatment lies in delivery. In the meantime, the aim is to monitor and control blood pressure and to plan delivery as close to fetal maturity as possible. Delivery is indicated if there is concern for maternal condition (e.g. as assessed by increasing blood pressure, deterioration in renal/liver function) or fetal condition (e.g. IUGR, fetal distress). The woman should be admitted to the antenatal ward and monitored to assess progression of the condition. Biochemical (renal and liver function) and haematological (to look for evidence of falling platelets or HELLP syndrome) assessment should be performed as described above. Regular (at least 4-hourly) blood pressure assessments should be made in order to identify worsening condition. A fluid balance chart should be commenced to identify oliguria, which again is associated with worsening of the condition. Twice daily urinalysis should be performed to assess increasing proteinuria. Assessment of fetal condition, including ultrasound biometry, umbilical Doppler and cardiotocography should be undertaken. Maternal steroids should be administered in case early delivery is indicated. Antihypertensive therapy should be commenced if the systolic blood pressure is >170 mmHg and the diastolic pressure is >110 mmHg. This controls blood pressure and reduces the risk of complications such as cerebrovascular accidents but does not alter the progression of pre-eclampsia. Labetalol and nifedipine are appropriate antihypertensive agents for this purpose. If there is hyperreflexia/clonus and/or HELLP syndrome, delivery is indicated. In this instance, magnesium sulphate as an anticonvulsant agent should be commenced to reduce the risk of eclampsia.

Box 5.1 Risks of pre-eclampsia

Maternal complications:
- Eclampsia.
- Cerebrovascular accident.
- HELLP syndrome.
- Disseminated intravascular coagulation.
- Liver failure.
- Renal failure.
- Pulmonary oedema.
- Maternal death.

Fetal complications:
- Intrauterine growth restriction.
- Placental abruption.
- Fetal death.

CASE 5.2 – I am 28 weeks pregnant and have sugar in my urine.

A1: What is the likely differential diagnosis?
- Reduced renal threshold for glucose during pregnancy.
- Gestational diabetes.

A2: What issues in the given history support the diagnosis?
The woman's age and her weight increase her risk of gestational diabetes.

A3: What additional features in the history would you seek to support a particular diagnosis?
Multiple pregnancy, a family history of diabetes in a first-degree relative, a previous history of gestational diabetes, a previous unexplained intrauterine death, polyhydramnios and a previous 'large-for-dates' (LFD) baby are all risk factors for gestational diabetes.

A4: What clinical examination would you perform and why?
Examination should include fundoscopy for diabetic retinopathy and abdominal palpation for evidence of a LFD fetus or polyhydramnios.

A5: What investigations would be most helpful and why?

● **Glucose tolerance test**	☑	A fasting blood glucose concentration >5.1 mmol/L and/or a 2-h blood glucose concentration >8.5 mmol/L using a 75 g carbohydrate test would confirm the diagnosis of gestational diabetes.
● **Glycated haemoglobin**	☑	To identify long-term hyperglycaemia.

A6: What treatment options are appropriate?

MANAGEMENT OF GESTATIONAL DIABETES
- Review of the woman's diet to include high levels of complex carbohydrate, soluble fibre and reduced saturated fats. An energy prescription of 30–35 kcal/kg pre-pregnant optimum body weight is ideal, with at least 50 per cent of energy being derived from carbohydrates.
- Pre-prandial blood glucose monitoring (i.e. four times daily) should be commenced. If blood glucose levels are consistently >6.0–7.0 mmol/L despite adherence to diet, either an oral hypoglycaemic agent, e.g. metformin, or insulin should be commenced. A regimen of pre-prandial short-acting insulin or analogue and overnight longer-acting insulin or analogue should be used. Insulin requirements will increase during pregnancy and should be adjusted accordingly.
- Measurement of glycated haemoglobin every 4–6 weeks is common practice, but has not been shown to improve outcome.
- A retinal examination should be performed every 4–6 weeks.

ANTENATAL CARE
- Ultrasound examination should be performed fortnightly in the third trimester to measure abdominal circumference as an assessment of fetal growth, to assess liquor volume and to perform umbilical arterial Doppler.
- More frequent visits will be necessary to allow optimal management of diabetic control and to screen for complications of pregnancy, which are more common (e.g. proteinuric hypertension).

- A multiprofessional team in a dedicated, well-organized, combined, diabetes antenatal clinic should assume responsibility for care. The team should include an obstetrician with an interest in diabetes in pregnancy, a diabetes physician, a midwife, a diabetes nurse and a dietitian.

TIMING AND MODE OF DELIVERY

- With good diabetic control and in the absence of obstetric complications, delivery at 38–9 weeks by the vaginal route should be the aim.
- Women with gestational diabetes who are on insulin require an insulin and dextrose infusion, aiming to keep blood sugar levels between 4.0 and 6.0 mmol/L. Blood glucose levels should be checked hourly. Women who are controlled by diet do not need to monitor blood glucose levels during labour.
- Effective pain relief is important and an epidural should be considered.
- Continual fetal heart rate monitoring should be used because of the increased risk of fetal distress.
- It is important to be aware of the increased risk of shoulder dystocia and to take appropriate precautions at delivery (i.e. maternal position [consider lithotomy] and episiotomy, particularly if the scans suggest that the fetus is LFD).

POSTNATAL CARE

- For women who are on metformin or insulin, this should be stopped after delivery of the placenta.
- Breast-feeding should be encouraged.
- All women with gestational diabetes should be seen at 6 weeks for a postnatal check and glucose tolerance test. In most women, this will be normal, but they remain at risk of developing diabetes in the future. This risk can be reduced by weight control and exercise. They should all therefore be given general advice about weight and diet, and should have annual fasting blood glucose tests for early detection of diabetes.

Box 5.2 Risks of gestational diabetes

Risks of gestational diabetes for the mother include:
- Macrosomia and a difficult delivery (shoulder dystocia or the need for caesarean section for cephalopelvic disproportion).
- Polyhydramnios.
- Risk of the mother developing diabetes in the future.

Risks of gestational diabetes for the baby include:
- Hypoglycaemia.
- Hypocalcaemia.
- Palsies.
- Fractures resulting from difficult delivery.

CASE 5.3 – I am pregnant and also anaemic.

A1: What is the likely differential diagnosis?

- Iron-deficiency anaemia.
- Sickle-cell disease.
- Thalassaemia.
- B_{12} or folate deficiency.

A2: What issues in the given history support the diagnosis?

Iron-deficiency anaemia is supported by the woman's high parity and narrow spacing between children. This is the most common type of anaemia in pregnancy, affecting about 10 per cent of women. Her vegetarian diet would predispose to reduced iron intake.

A3: What additional features in the history would you seek to support a particular diagnosis?

An additional history would include symptoms (e.g. tiredness, breathlessness, 'light-headedness' or 'dizziness'), evidence of chronic blood loss (e.g. menorrhagia), a previous history of anaemia, the use of iron supplements and the patient's country of origin. Symptoms of anaemia are usually absent unless the haemoglobin concentration is <8 g/dL. Around 10 per cent of African Caribbean individuals in the UK are heterozygous for sickle-cell disease, and thalassaemia is most prevalent in individuals from the Mediterranean region and south-east Asia.

A4: What clinical examination would you perform and why?

Examination would include a search for evidence of pallor (generally the sclera and palms) and abdominal examination for hepatosplenomegaly.

A5: What investigations would be most helpful and why?

• **Blood film**	✓	Microcytosis and hypochromia can be seen on blood film in iron-deficiency anaemia. Hypersegmented neutrophils are seen in folate deficiency.
• **FBC**	✓	Both mean cell volume (MCV) and mean cell haemoglobin (MCH) are reduced in iron-deficiency anaemia. MCV is usually increased in folate deficiency. Haemoglobin estimation in pregnancy should not be the only parameter to be assessed as a sign of anaemia because it can be lowered as a result of haemodilution. If the MCV is in the normal range, this would signify haemodilution; if microcytosis is present, an iron deficiency or haemoglobinopathy is likely.
• **B_{12} and folate levels**	✓	If blood film is macrocytic.
• **Transferrin, iron and total iron binding capacity**	✓	If microcytosis is present.

- **Ferritin levels** ☑ Ferritin levels should be measured if microcytosis is present. Levels are reduced in iron-deficiency anaemia.

- **Red cell folate** ± Red cell folate should be measured if anaemia is present without marked microcytosis.

- **Sickledex test and haemoglobin electrophoresis** ± Sickledex test and if positive haemoglobin electrophoresis for sickle-cell trait. If the woman is Sickledex positive, her partner should be tested and appropriate counselling given about the prenatal diagnosis.

- **Haemoglobin A$_2$** ± Haemoglobin A$_2$ quantitation is required for thalassaemia and, again if a positive result is obtained, the partner should be tested.

A6: What treatment options are appropriate?

- Iron-deficiency anaemia should be treated with iron supplementation. Initially this should be oral (e.g. ferrous sulphate), but if not tolerated by the patient can be given by intravenous infusion (Venofer). The rarer folate and B$_{12}$ deficiencies should be treated with appropriate supplements. The aim should be to correct anaemia before delivery. However, as folic acid reduces the risk of neural tube defects, it should be recommended to all women.

- Heterozygous sickle-cell carriers usually have no problems and do not require treatment. They may in extreme situations (e.g. hypoxia, infections) develop 'crises'. Homozygote carriers are likely to have been affected by 'crises' and have chronic haemolytic anaemia all their lives. In pregnancy, they have increased perinatal mortality and are at risk of thrombosis, infection and sickle 'crises'. Treatment includes exchange transfusions, screening for infection, folic acid and avoidance of precipitating factors for crises. Iron should be avoided.

- For women with heterozygous α-thalassaemia, iron and folate supplementation are required. In β-thalassaemia, heterozygous women have a chronic anaemia that can worsen during pregnancy. They may require transfusion. Pregnancy in homozygous individuals is uncommon. In these cases, folic acid is required, but iron should be avoided.

ᴬᴬ OSCE counselling cases

OSCE COUNSELLING CASE 5.1 – **I have diabetes and want to become pregnant.**

A1: What pre-pregnancy counselling would you provide for this woman?

- The diabetic control should be optimized before pregnancy in order to reduce the risk of congenital anomalies. If the patient is not regularly monitoring her blood sugar levels, this would need to be commenced with the aim of adjusting insulin to keep pre-prandial levels to between 4 and 7 mmol/L. A glycated haemoglobin concentration would give an indication of longer-term control and should ideally be <7 per cent before conceiving.
- The provision of glucagon would need to be checked because of the increased risk of hypoglycaemic attacks with the tighter control. It would be important for the woman's partner to know when and how to administer the glucagon.
- Commence folic acid supplementation (5 mg daily) to reduce the risk of neural tube defects and aspirin (75 mg daily) to reduce the risk of pre-eclampsia.
- Check whether the woman is rubella immune and give immunization before stopping contraception, if she is not.
- Emphasize the need to report early after a missed period to ensure early referral to a specialist multidisciplinary antenatal clinic.
- Arrange an eye examination to identify pre-existing retinopathy, which should be treated before pregnancy.

OSCE COUNSELLING CASE 5.2 – **I have epilepsy and I want to become pregnant.**

A1: What pre-pregnancy care and counselling would you give this woman?

- Most babies who are born to mothers with epilepsy are normal. However, women with epilepsy, particularly those taking antiepileptic drugs, are at increased risk of giving birth to a baby with congenital anomalies (e.g. neural tube defects).
- Before and during pregnancy, the aim should be to prescribe the lowest dose and number of antiepileptic drugs necessary to protect against seizures. Suggest referral to a neurologist to consider pre-pregnancy withdrawal of antiepileptic drugs or a change to monotherapy.
- Emphasize the importance of periconceptual folic acid.
- Recommend a detailed ultrasound scan at 18–20 weeks to identify fetal anomalies.
- Check whether the woman is rubella immune and provide immunization, if appropriate.

REVISION PANEL

- HELLP (haemolysis, elevated liver enzymes, low platelets) syndrome is associated with impending eclampsia in women with pre-eclampsia.
- Gestational diabetes is associated with a high risk of type 2 diabetes in later life. This risk can be significantly reduced by lifestyle (diet and exercise) changes.
- Optimal control of diabetes periconceptually and during pregnancy reduces the risks of pregnancy-associated complications. Folic acid should be given at 5 mg dose to reduce the risk of neural tube defects and low dose aspirin should be commenced at 8–12 weeks to reduce the risk of pre-eclampsia.
- The only 'cure' for pre-eclampsia is delivery of the fetus and placenta.

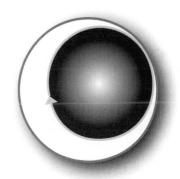

⑥ Puerperium

Questions

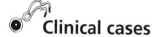

Clinical cases

For each of the case scenarios given, consider the following:

Q1: What is the likely differential diagnosis?
Q2: What issues in the given history support the diagnosis?
Q3: What additional features in the history would you seek to support a particular diagnosis?
Q4: What clinical examination would you perform and why?
Q5: What investigations would be most helpful and why?
Q6: What treatment options are appropriate?

CASE 6.1 – My baby has just been delivered and I am bleeding heavily.

A 36-year-old woman with five children and a history of previous short labours delivered her baby 10 min ago. She had been in labour on this occasion for 12 h after a spontaneous onset. She continues to bleed heavily.

CASE 6.2 – I had a baby 3 days ago and feel shivery.

A 34-year-old primiparous woman had a traumatic vaginal delivery after an 18-h labour. Labour was induced after pre-labour rupture of the membranes for over 48 h. Three days post-delivery, the woman feels shivery and has had a temperature of 38.4 °C and 38.5 °C measured 4 h apart. She is a smoker, but had stopped smoking during pregnancy.

CASE 6.3 – The midwife is concerned because I have little interest in my baby.

An older primigravida feels that she has very little interest in her baby 3 days after delivery. She is a solicitor by profession and became pregnant after assisted conception. The pregnancy and delivery were uneventful. There is no past history or family history of mental illness.

ÅÅ OSCE counselling cases

OSCE COUNSELLING CASE 6.1 – **Should I be breast-feeding my baby?**

A primigravida has just delivered a healthy 3600 g baby.

Q1: What are the advantages and disadvantages of breast-feeding?

OSCE COUNSELLING CASE 6.2 – **My baby has breathing difficulties after a caesarean birth.**

A baby has been admitted to the neonatal unit with breathing difficulties after a caesarean section at term because of failure to progress. There was no fetal distress or birth asphyxia. The baby started grunting at 30 min of age. Clinical examination and radiograph suggest transient tachypnoea of the newborn (TTN).

Q1: Explain to the mother what is wrong with her baby and how it will be managed.

Answers

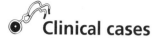

Clinical cases

CASE 6.1 – My baby has just been delivered and I am bleeding heavily.

A1: What is the likely differential diagnosis?

Primary postpartum haemorrhage:
- Atonic uterus, with or without retained placenta or placental segments.
- Cervical, vaginal or perineal trauma.

A2: What issues in the given history support the diagnosis?

Grand multiparity and prolonged labour are both risk factors for atonic postpartum haemorrhage.

A3: What additional features in the history would you seek to support a particular diagnosis?

A history of induced labour, retained placenta, previous postpartum haemorrhage, surgical delivery, polyhydramnios, multiple pregnancy, antepartum haemorrhage, previous caesarean section and a coagulation defect would all increase this woman's risk of postpartum haemorrhage.

A4: What clinical examination would you perform and why?

Examination would include measurement of pulse and blood pressure for evidence of shock. An assessment of blood loss and continuing loss is required. Abdominal examination would include palpation of the uterine fundus to identify a poorly contracted uterus. A check for obvious vaginal/perineal trauma should be made and the midwife should be asked to check the completeness of the placenta.

A5: What investigations would be most helpful and why?

• **FBC**	✓	To identify anaemia and platelet count.
• **Blood cross-match**	✓	To replace blood loss and treat shock.
• **Clotting screen**	✓	To identify a coagulopathy.

A6: What treatment options are appropriate?

- Initial management should be to obtain intravenous access (two wide bore Venflons) and commence intravenous fluids. The uterine fundus should be 'rubbed up' if it is not contracted. An intravenous oxytocin (Syntocinon) infusion should be commenced and intramuscular/intravenous ergometrine given to contract the uterus. Any vaginal or perineal trauma should be sutured.
- If the bleeding continues, manage shock and call for senior obstetric and anaesthetic assistance. Give oxygen and commence colloid and/or blood when cross-matched, or O-negative blood. Ensure that an adequate request has been made for cross-matched blood (at least 8 units) and check clotting. Continue to compress the uterus bimanually if it is not contracted. Continue the intravenous infusion of Syntocinon. Consider giving rectal, intramuscular or intramyometrial prostaglandin. Catheterize the patient to monitor urine output and insert a central venous pressure line. If the bleeding persists,

examine under an anaesthetic to check that the uterine cavity is empty of retained products of conception, and to identify and suture any trauma to the cervix, vagina or perineum. If bleeding still persists, consider a Rusch balloon, B-Lynch suture, interventional radiology to embolize uterine arteries or laparotomy with ligation of the internal iliac arteries or hysterectomy.

CASE 6.2 – I had a baby 3 days ago and feel shivery.

A1: What is the likely differential diagnosis?

- Endometritis.
- Perineal wound infection.
- Breast infection/abscess.
- Urinary tract infection (UTI).
- Chest infection.
- Deep venous thrombosis (DVT).

A2: What issues in the given history support the diagnosis?

Symptoms of shivers and a temperature are suggestive of an infection. Perineal lacerations and episiotomies can become infected. A prolonged labour with ruptured membranes and repeated vaginal examinations during induction of labour can result in endometritis. Smoking is a risk factor for chest infection. A maternal pyrexia of >38 °C is not usually associated with deep venous thrombosis, which causes a low-grade pyrexia.

A3: What additional features in the history would you seek to support a particular diagnosis?

For endometritis, the lochia may be offensive. A history of frequency and dysuria may indicate a UTI, which is a common cause of postpartum pyrexia. If the patient is also catheterized during labour, this can lead to a UTI. An enquiry should be made to ensure that the placenta was complete at the third stage of labour, to exclude infection of a retained placenta. This history may not be diagnostic.

A4: What clinical examination would you perform and why?

Pulse, blood pressure, peripheral perfusion and signs of cyanosis should be sought. Examination is required of the chest, breasts (enlargement, warmth and tenderness and a fluctuant tender mass, together with enlarged axillary lymph nodes may be caused by an abscess), abdomen (to check for involution of the uterus), loins (for renal tenderness), and intravenous access sites and legs (for swelling and tenderness). Vulval examination of the perineal wound is also indicated. A vaginal examination should also be performed to determine whether the cervical os is open. It may indicate retained products and an enlarged tender uterus. If the patient had a caesarean section, a wound haematoma infection or abscess would need to be excluded.

A5: What investigations would be most helpful and why?

• **FBC**	✓	Blood for white cell count – increased polymorphs would indicate infection.
• **CRP**	✓	
• **HVS and endocervical swabs**	✓	For culture and sensitivity testing for infection.
• **Urine culture**	✓	To exclude a UTI.

- **Blood cultures** ☑ To exclude septicaemia in view of the patient's high temperature.
- **Chest radiograph** ☑ To exclude a chest infection if clinical signs.
- **Ultrasound Doppler of leg/pelvic veins** ☑ To exclude a DVT if clinical signs.

A6: What treatment options are appropriate?

- Endometritis: co-amoxiclav (Augmentin) and metronidazole or erythromycin and metronidazole (covers anaerobes).
- Urinary tract infection: cephalosporins, penicillins/co-amoxiclav (Augmentin) (covers Gram-negative cocci). Increase fluid intake.
- Perineal wound infection: administer broad-spectrum antibiotics, which should include metronidazole. Keep the wound clean and dry to allow rapid healing. If an abscess is present, any sutures should be cut to allow the abscess to drain.
- Breast infection/abscess: stop breast-feeding from the affected breast, but still continue to express the milk. Administer penicillins/broad-spectrum antibiotics. Incise and drain if there is an obvious abscess.
- Chest infection: chest physiotherapy, and amoxicillin/co-amoxiclav (Augmentin) (covers Gram-positive cocci).
- Deep venous thrombosis: low molecular weight heparin, e.g. Fragmin.

Management of DVT should be arranged in collaboration with the physicians so that the appropriate anticoagulant regimen is administered. Risk markers should be tested 6 weeks postpartum (i.e. protein S and C deficiency, factor V Leiden mutation and anti-thrombin III levels).

CASE 6.3 – **The midwife is concerned because I have little interest in my baby.**

A1: What is the likely differential diagnosis?

- Postpartum 'baby blues'.
- Depression.
- Puerperal psychosis.

A2: What issues in the given history support the diagnosis?

In most cases with the given history, there is no psychiatric problem because minor psychological symptoms are common after birth. Postpartum 'baby blues' are at their worst around days 3–5 after the birth, but resolve by about day 10. However, this case needs further investigation in order to exclude major psychosis or depression, particularly if the symptoms occur later, around 4–6 weeks after birth. Lack of family history and past history of mental illness support a benign transient phenomenon, but the woman's age, higher social class, primigravidity and infertility treatment are all risk factors for major mental illness.

A3: What additional features in the history would you seek to support a particular diagnosis?

The history should explore psychological symptoms such as variation in mood, poor sleep, weeping, lethargy, irritability, hallucinations, delusions, etc. Operative mode of delivery, multiple pregnancy and complications during pregnancy all increase the likelihood of major mental illness.

A4: What clinical examination would you perform and why?

A mental state examination is required.

A5: What investigations would be most helpful and why?

● **TFT**	✓	Thyrotoxicosis should be excluded if major mental illness is suspected.

A6: What treatment options are appropriate?

- Postpartum blues: psychological support and reassurance should be offered.
- Refer the patient to a psychiatrist if depression or psychosis is suspected. Early diagnosis is important, because it can interfere with mother–baby bonding.
- Depression: antidepressants (e.g. imipramine, which does not interfere with breast-feeding).
- Puerperal psychosis: admission to a psychiatric ward is essential, because there is a risk of suicide. The mother should be separated from the baby because there is a risk of neglect and harm. Neuroleptics may be used.

ⅲⅲ OSCE counselling cases

OSCE COUNSELLING CASE 6.1 – **Should I be breast-feeding my baby?**

A1: What are the advantages and disadvantages of breast-feeding?

Advantages include:
- No cost.
- No risk of infection from bottles.
- Breast milk contains protein, fat and solute content 'designed' for babies (i.e. appropriate nutritional content).
- Contraceptive when fully breast-feeding.
- Provides protection against infection (by providing passive immunity via maternal antibodies) and allergies in neonate.
- Reduced respiratory and gastrointestinal illness in the child.
- Infant–mother bonding promoted.
- Protection against maternal breast, endometrial and ovarian cancer.
- Rapid reduction in maternal weight gained from pregnancy.
- Effect on child development (e.g. potentially improved cognitive function).

Disadvantages include:
- Breast milk jaundice is more common.
- Can lead to maternal exhaustion because it involves feeding on demand.
- Can cause pain/discomfort as a result of breast engorgement.
- Leaking of milk from breasts may occur.
- Without good support/encouragement, particularly in the early days when establishing breast-feeding, there is a greater likelihood of giving up because of poor milk flow.

Despite these minor disadvantages, all mothers should be encouraged to breast-feed their babies.

OSCE COUNSELLING CASE 6.2 – **My baby has breathing difficulties after a caesarean birth.**

A1: Explain to the mother what is wrong with her baby and how it will be managed.

Transient tachypnoea of the newborn:
- A benign transient problem with recovery within 1–2 days.
- A problem of retained lung fluid.
- Managed with supportive treatment such as oxygen and intravenous fluids.
- Antibiotics can be prescribed, but are not always necessary.
- There are no long-term sequelae.
- The differential diagnosis is of either infection or respiratory distress syndrome.

REVISION PANEL

- Grand multiparity, prolonged labour, polyhydramnios and multiple pregnancy are risk factors for atoric postpartum haemorrhage.
- The latest confidential enquiry into maternal deaths identified genital tract infection as being the leading direct cause of death. Evidence of infection in the puerperium must therefore be monitored closely and treated early and appropriately.
- All women should be considered post-partum for DVT risk and commenced on appropriate prophylaxis depending on that risk.

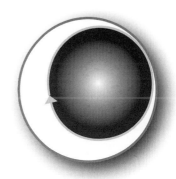

7 Abnormal uterine bleeding

Questions

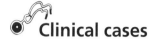

Clinical cases

For each of the case scenarios given, consider the following:

> **Q1**: What is the likely differential diagnosis?
> **Q2**: What issues in the given history support the diagnosis?
> **Q3**: What additional features in the history would you seek to support a particular diagnosis?
> **Q4**: What clinical examination would you perform and why?
> **Q5**: What investigations would be most helpful and why?
> **Q6**: What treatment options are appropriate?

CASE 7.1 – **My periods are regular but heavy.**

A 36-year-old nulliparous woman presents to the gynaecology outpatient clinic with heavy, regular periods. Her menstrual cycle is 28 days. The periods last for 5 days, with clots during the first 2 days. Up to 20 sanitary towels and supersize tampons are required for each period. The patient has no significant dysmenorrhoea and there is no intermenstrual bleeding. She complains of feeling 'run down' and lacking in energy. Her recent smear was negative and she is not using any contraception.

CASE 7.2 – **My periods are heavy and irregular.**

A 47-year-old schoolteacher with two children complains of a 9-month history of heavy irregular periods. Her menstrual cycle is erratic and can vary between 3 and 6 weeks, with periods lasting 5–7 days. Before the onset of menstrual problems her cycles were regular (every 4 weeks). Her recent cervical smear is negative, and she has no intermenstrual bleeding. The patient has been sterilized.

CASE 7.3 – **I have vaginal bleeding after intercourse.**

A 32-year-old woman presents with a 6-month history of bleeding after intercourse. She is uncertain about when her last smear was taken. She has four children and currently uses the combined oral contraceptive pill for contraception.

👫 OSCE counselling cases

OSCE COUNSELLING CASE 7.1 – **Should I have surgery for heavy periods?**

A 45-year-old woman presents with an 18-month history of increasingly heavy periods. She has a regular cycle with 7 days of bleeding every 28–30 days. Clinical examination and investigations are unremarkable. A diagnosis of dysfunctional uterine bleeding (DUB) is made.

Q1: If she opted for surgical management, what factors would you consider important when counselling her?

OSCE COUNSELLING CASE 7.2 – **Will hysterectomy affect my sex life?**

A 44-year-old woman is having considerable problems with heavy menstrual bleeding (DUB), which has been unresponsive to medical treatment. She has been offered a hysterectomy by her gynaecologist, who has given her some time to consider this option. She mentioned this to a friend, who told her that the operation 'ruins your sex life and makes you incontinent'.

Q1: Can you reassure her? What factors would you consider important when counselling her?

Key concepts

In order to work through the core clinical cases in this chapter, you will need to understand the following key concepts.

MENORRHAGIA

The preferred term is now heavy menstrual bleeding (HMB). Excessive loss of blood during menstruation is objectively measured to be >80 mL. In practice, this definition is seldom used and the effect of heavy menstruation on the patient's quality of life is considered to be more important.

- Dysfunctional uterine bleeding (DUB) is classified when there is no organic disease of the genital tract. It accounts for two-thirds of all heavy menstrual bleeding cases. It can be anovular or more commonly ovular, i.e. with a regular cycle.
- Heavy menstrual bleeding can also be caused by bleeding disorders such as idiopathic thrombocytopenia (ITP), von Willebrand's disease (factor VIII deficiency) or anticoagulation therapy (uncommon).

DYSMENORRHOEA

Painful menstrual periods:

- Primary: not associated with organic disease of the genital tract or a psychological cause.
- Secondary: a cause can be found, e.g. endometriosis, chronic pelvic inflammatory disease (PID).

PREMENSTRUAL SYNDROME

Recurrent somatic, psychological or behavioural symptoms occurring in the premenstrual phase and up to the point of menses. They produce social, family and occupational disturbance, usually relieved by menstruation.

Answers

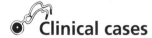 **Clinical cases**

CASE 7.1 – **My periods are regular but heavy.**

A1: What is the likely differential diagnosis?

- Ovular DUB.
- Uterine leiomyoma (fibroids).
- Adenomyosis is a form of uterine endometriosis where the endometriosis is found in the myometrium.
- Secondary to other causes, i.e. ITP, von Willebrand's disease.

A2: What issues in the given history support the diagnosis?

HMB is commonly associated with ovular DUB or fibroids. Anovular DUB would lengthen the cycle and is more common in perimenopausal women (see Case 7.2). Intermenstrual bleeding could be associated with anovular DUB, endometrial or cervical polyp or, very rarely, carcinoma, but highly unlikely at this age. Clots and the large number of sanitary towels and tampons required indicate the severity of the problem. Painful periods (dysmenorrhoea) could indicate endometriosis or adenomyosis.

A3: What additional features in the history would you seek to support a particular diagnosis?

Indications for the quality of life (e.g. effect on social life, days off work, sexual relationships, family life) to establish the severity of the problem. Enquire about drug history and family history of bleeding disorders.

A4: What clinical examination would you perform and why?

Pallor on general examination may indicate anaemia caused by blood loss. Bimanual pelvic examination should be undertaken to assess uterine size, mobility and uterine fibroids. Uterine tenderness/bogginess would indicate a suspicion of adenomyosis.

A5: What investigations would be most helpful and why?

• **FBC**	✓	To exclude iron-deficiency anaemia (indicated by low mean cell volume [MCV]).
• **TFT**	✗	Not required as a routine investigation.
• **USS**	±	Can give the position, size and number of fibroids or show normal pelvic viscera (DUB).
• **Endometrial biopsy**	✗	Only essential in women over 45 years of age because in premenopausal women <45 years the risk of endometrial cancer is extremely low (<4:100 000). It may be undertaken in younger women with menorrhagia who are not responding to medical treatment.

A6: What treatment options are appropriate?

SUPPORTIVE

If investigations are normal, reassure the patient about the absence of pathology. Treat anaemia with therapeutic doses of iron supplements. Compliance can be assessed by asking about dark stools. Iron therapy itself can improve quality of life.

MEDICAL

- Tranexamic acid taken during the menses is the first-line treatment of choice. It will reduce menstrual blood loss by approximately 50 per cent.
- Mefenamic acid is useful if there is associated pain. It can be used in conjunction with tranexamic acid.
- Combined oral contraceptive pill, only if risk factors have been excluded, i.e. smoking, raised body mass index, diabetes, hypertension.
- Levonorgestrel intrauterine system (LNG-IUS) – warn of irregularity of menstrual cycle, which can last up to 9 months.
- Progestogens should be used in high doses throughout the cycle. It is ineffective when used in low doses and in the second half of the menstrual cycle. Primarily used for anovular DUB (see Case 7.2).
- Danazol – should not be used due to side effects such as acne, weight gain and voice changes.

SURGICAL

- Not applicable to this patient because her family is *not* complete.
- Endometrial ablation when the family is complete. There are several different types available, e.g. first-generation resection or rollerball and second-generation global endometrial ablation devices such as hot water, microwave or bipolar energy sources. They all have a success rate of approximately 80 per cent. Success rates depend on uterine size and presence of fibroids and adenomyosis.
- In cases of submucous fibroids (Fig. 7.1), hysteroscopic myomectomy of the submucous component only would be suitable if fertility is to be preserved. Success rate is approximately 80 per cent. Treatment of subserosal or intramural fibroids does not usually result in appreciable menstrual loss improvement.
- Hysterectomy (abdominal, laparoscopic, subtotal or vaginal) is definitive, if the family is complete.

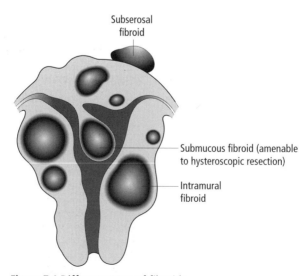

Subserosal fibroid

Submucous fibroid (amenable to hysteroscopic resection)

Intramural fibroid

Figure 7.1 Different types of fibroids.

CASE 7.2 – **My periods are heavy and irregular.**

A1: What is the likely differential diagnosis?

- Anovular DUB.
- Endometrial pathology (e.g. hyperplasia).
- Climacteric (period of 2–3 years before menopause).
- Fibroids/adenomyosis.
- Ovarian pathology.

A2: What issues in the given history support the diagnosis?

Perimenopausal women have failing ovarian function and this, associated with an irregularity of the oestrogen/progesterone balance, gives rise to an irregular cycle. In anovular DUB, unopposed high oestrogen levels can cause a prolonged cycle in which the endometrium undergoes hyperplasia (endometrial glands are dilated and crowded). The duration of symptoms is an indication that this condition is unlikely to resolve spontaneously without treatment.

A3: What additional features in the history would you seek to support a particular diagnosis?

Menopausal symptoms of hot flushes, night sweats, loss of libido and dry skin associated with the climacteric should be sought. Obesity, hypertension and diabetes are risk factors for hyperplasia and endometrial cancer.

A4: What clinical examination would you perform and why?

General examination to exclude pallor. Abdominal examination to exclude pelvic mass secondary to fibroids. Bimanual examination to assess uterine size/mobility and adnexal pathology. This would exclude fibroids and ovarian pathology.

A5: What investigations would be most helpful and why?

● **FBC**	✓	To exclude iron-deficiency anaemia.
● **FSH**	±	To check for ovarian function, if there are any menopausal symptoms. Gonadotrophin levels such as follicle-stimulating hormone (FSH) levels should be measured during or just after menses.
● **USS**	✓	To exclude uterine and ovarian pathology. Endometrial thickness indicates endometrial pathology. Uterine fibroids or adnexal masses may be visualized.
● **Outpatient hysteroscopy**	✓	To exclude endometrial polyps/submucous fibroids.
● **Outpatient endometrial biopsy**	✓	Endometrial biopsy is the definitive way to exclude hyperplasia and carcinoma of the endometrium. It is recommended that all women over 45 years of age with irregular vaginal bleeding should have an endometrial biopsy. Outpatient biopsy is diagnostic of detecting endometrial pathology when it is present and should be used wherever possible instead of inpatient general anaesthetic biopsy (D&C).

A6: What treatment options are appropriate?

SUPPORTIVE

Treat anaemia with iron supplements.

MEDICAL

- If the patient is in the climacteric (perimenopausal), combined hormone replacement therapy may be prescribed (see Case 8.3 and OSCE Counselling Case 8.1).
- Progestogens in high doses throughout the cycle.
- With anovular DUB that has resulted in endometrial hyperplasia (without atypia), progestogen treatment is required in a continuous high-dose manner.
- Consider using a levonorgestrel intrauterine system, which has the advantage of releasing continuous progestogens locally in the uterus for up to 5 years.

SURGICAL

- Hysterectomy (abdominal, laparoscopic, subtotal or vaginal) is definitive. When hyperplasia is associated with cellular atypia, total hysterectomy with bilateral salpingo-oophorectomy is mandatory.

CASE 7.3 – I have vaginal bleeding after intercourse.

A1: What is the likely differential diagnosis?

- Cervical ectropion.
- Cervical polyp.
- Cervicitis.
- Cervical carcinoma.

A2: What issues in the given history support the diagnosis?

The pill is associated with cervical ectropion. The pill together with pregnancy and puberty are risk factors that are commonly remembered as the three Ps.

A3: What additional features in the history would you seek to support a particular diagnosis?

It would be important to ascertain this woman's social status, her employment, sexual history (age at first intercourse, number of sexual partners) and whether she is a smoker because all of these are risk factors for a cervical abnormality such as dyskaryosis or cervical carcinoma. A vaginal discharge may be associated with cervicitis.

A4: What clinical examination would you perform and why?

A careful inspection of the vulva and speculum examination of the vagina and particularly the cervix is mandatory. (See Case 12.1 for details of examination in cases of vaginal discharge.)

A5: What investigations would be most helpful and why?

● **Cervical**	✓	Obtain report of last smear, or take one if there is no bleeding at speculum smear examination.
● **Vaginal or cervical swabs for microscopy and culture**	±	Only if infection is suspected or in cases associated with vaginal discharge.

- **Colposcopy and cervical biopsies** $\boxed{\pm}$ Mandatory if there is any suspicion of malignancy or if cervical smear result is abnormal.
- **Hysteroscopy** $\boxed{x}$ Only necessary if there was associated persistent intermenstrual bleeding, indicating the possibility of an endometrial polyp.

A6: What treatment options are appropriate?

SUPPORTIVE
Reassure the patient if there is no pathology.

MEDICAL
Infection should be treated with appropriate antibiotics according to the results of culture and sensitivity reports.

SURGICAL
- If a polyp is evident, this should be avulsed and sent for histopathological assessment. This can be done as an outpatient procedure without anaesthesia.
- Cervical ablation: if the smear is normal, a cervical ectropion can be reasonably treated in the outpatient clinic (e.g. with cryotherapy, cold coagulation, laser or large loop excision of the transformation zone – LLETZ).

👥 OSCE counselling cases

OSCE COUNSELLING CASE 7.1 – **Should I have surgery for heavy periods?**

A1: If she opted for surgical management, what factors would you consider important when counselling her?

The surgical approaches that are available (i.e. endometrial ablation or hysterectomy):
- Second-generation endometrial ablation can be carried out in the outpatient setting, using local anaesthesia. The success rate is approximately 80 per cent, but amenorrhoea is not guaranteed. There is a possibility that a hysterectomy may be required at the time of surgery if a complication arises, particularly with first-generation techniques, or at a later date if ablation is not successful. In addition, pregnancy should be avoided and sterilization may be considered at the same time as ablation. Recovery rates are short.
- If a hysterectomy is decided on, consideration would need to be given to the route, i.e. vaginal, abdominal or laparoscopically-assisted. If abdominal, whether this would be total or subtotal. Consideration should be given to whether the ovaries should be removed in order to reduce the risk of future ovarian cancer. Oestrogen-alone hormone replacement treatment may be required, but combined HRT is needed in subtotal hysterectomy. Risk of ovarian cancer is low if there is no family history.
- Hysterectomy recovery rates are reducing with the introduction of enhanced recovery methods, i.e. early mobilization, early introduction of diet, early discharge, which lead to full recovery as early as 3–4 weeks, rather than the traditional 6–12 weeks.

OSCE COUNSELLING CASE 7.2 – **Will hysterectomy affect my sex life?**

A1: Can you reassure her? What factors would you consider important when counselling her?

- Bladder function: the bladder innervation may be altered, but evidence of an increased incidence of incontinence is conflicting.
- Bowel function: again there is conflicting evidence, with some studies suggesting an increase in the incidence of irritable bowel syndrome and constipation, and others showing no change.
- Sexual function: both psychological and physical factors influence sexual function. It is generally accepted that sexual function remains unchanged and may even improve as the inherent problem of heavy periods has been resolved. There is no benefit in performing subtotal hysterectomy in terms of preserving sexual function.

REVISION PANEL

- For clinical purposes, HMB should be defined as excessive menstrual blood loss, which interferes with the woman's physical, emotional, social and material quality of life, and which can occur alone or in combination with other symptoms. Any interventions should aim to improve quality of life measures rather than focusing on menstrual blood loss.
- Therapeutic iron supplements alone can significantly improve quality of life.
- In premenopausal women, the risk of endometrial cancer is extremely low, but endometrial hyperplasia has to be excluded.
- In women with HMB alone, with a uterus no bigger than a 10-week pregnancy, endometrial ablation should be considered preferable to hysterectomy.
- Although hysterectomy is a definitive option for heavy menstrual bleeding, it should not be offered as first-line treatment unless gross disease is present, e.g. large multiple fibroids.

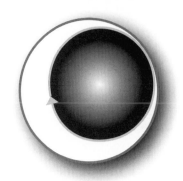

8 Amenorrhoea and menopause

Questions

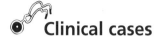

Clinical cases

For each of the case scenarios given, consider the following:

> **Q1**: What is the likely differential diagnosis?
> **Q2**: What issues in the given history support the diagnosis?
> **Q3**: What additional features in the history would you seek to support a particular diagnosis?
> **Q4**: What clinical examination would you perform and why?
> **Q5**: What investigations would be most helpful and why?
> **Q6**: What treatment options are appropriate?

CASE 8.1 – **My periods are infrequent. I have not had any for 7 months.**

A 26-year-old woman attends a gynaecology clinic concerned that she has not had a menstrual period for 7 months. She had her first period when she was 12 years old. Her periods have been gradually becoming more infrequent. She keeps athletically fit and has recently been training for a marathon and has lost some weight. She has a normal healthy appetite and diet. She claims not to have been sexually active for the past 12 months. Her home pregnancy test is negative.

CASE 8.2 – **I have intolerable menstrual periods.**

A 35-year-old woman has been experiencing pelvic pain, irritability, bloatedness and breast pain for 3–4 days before her periods. These symptoms have occurred cyclically over a period of 4–6 months and they disappear after the onset of menses. Her periods are regular and painful but not heavy. She has two children and uses condoms for contraception. There is no history of psychiatric illness.

CASE 8.3 – **Should I take HRT (hormone replacement therapy)?**

A slim 52-year-old university lecturer presents with an 18-month history of amenorrhoea and a 3-year history of hot flushes and night sweats. She has a family history of heart disease and breast cancer.

👫 OSCE counselling cases

OSCE COUNSELLING CASE 8.1 – **HRT compliance.**

A 48-year-old woman has menopausal symptoms. As a result of this and the fact that she has a family history of osteoporosis, she wishes to start HRT. However, compliance is a problem in women who start HRT.

Q1: What issues should be considered for improving this woman's compliance?

Q2: What would be an appropriate screening programme for this patient if she were happy to start HRT?

OSCE COUNSELLING CASE 8.2 – **Controversies with HRT.**

A 54-year-old has been told that she should stop taking her combined HRT because this is associated with an increased risk of breast cancer. She has enjoyed the HRT benefits and does not want to stop treatment.

Q1: What are the benefits and risks of HRT in the light of current evidence?

Q2: How can the HRT preparation be altered to suit her so that she can continue using HRT?

🔑 Key concepts

In order to work through the core clinical cases in this chapter, you will need to understand the following key concepts.

PUBERTY

- Time of onset of ovulatory and endocrine ovarian function, making an individual capable of reproduction.
- Delayed puberty is a lack of secondary sexual characteristics by the age of 14 years.

AMENORRHOEA

Lack of menstruation (this is a symptom, not a diagnosis).
- Primary: lack of menstruation by 16 years of age in a girl with normal growth and secondary sexual characteristics.
- Secondary: amenorrhoea for 6 months or for a duration of more than three times the length of previous menstrual cycles after an individual has formerly had menstrual periods.

OLIGOMENORRHOEA

Infrequent periods with a menstrual cycle longer than 35 days.

MENOPAUSE

Lack of menstruation for more than 12 months, associated with cessation of ovarian function and reproductive capacity.

PREMATURE MENOPAUSE

Menopause before the age of 35 years.

HIRSUTISM

Excessive growth of sexual (androgen-dependent) hairs.

VIRILISM

Androgenic changes more extensive than hirsutism, including amenorrhoea, breast atrophy, clitoromegaly and temporal balding.

Answers

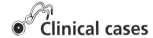 Clinical cases

CASE 8.1 – **My periods are infrequent. I have not had any for 7 months.**

A1: What is the likely differential diagnosis?

- Secondary amenorrhoea:
  - stress-related amenorrhoea;
  - polycystic ovarian syndrome (PCOS);
  - hyperprolactinaemia;
  - hyper-/hypothyroidism.
- Premature menopause.

A2: What issues in the given history support the diagnosis?

Pregnancy, the most common cause of secondary amenorrhoea, is unlikely in this case because the patient is not sexually active and a urinary pregnancy test is negative. Although she normally keeps fit, the excessive recent training over and above her normal routine level of fitness is likely to be a possible cause of her amenorrhoea. Moreover, as she has a normal diet, she does not have anorexia nervosa-related amenorrhoea.

A3: What additional features in the history would you seek to support a particular diagnosis?

An additional history should be obtained about menopausal symptoms (i.e. hot flushes, night sweats), in order to exclude premature menopause. Precise information about weight loss will be helpful because sudden excessive loss of >10kg is associated with amenorrhoea. PCOS would normally be associated with infertility and oligomenorrhoea. Headaches and visual disturbances may suggest pressure on the optic chiasma from a prolactinoma in the anterior pituitary. Symptoms of intolerance of extremes of temperature, feeling very energetic or lethargic, and excessive weight loss or weight gain would be consistent with hyper-/hypothyroidism. A drug history (e.g. progestogens and major tranquillizers such as phenothiazines) is associated with a lack of menstruation.

A4: What clinical examination would you perform and why?

The patient's weight should be measured (this may not be diagnostic, but it will be helpful in management and follow-up). The condition of the skin and hair may indicate thyroid abnormalities. Hirsutism and acne are associated with PCOS. Evidence of striae and stigmata of virilization may be an indication of severe PCOS or a hormone-producing tumour. The visual fields should be examined in cases of prolactinoma. A breast examination should be performed to ensure normality of secondary sexual characteristics and to check for galactorrhoea (a sign of prolactinoma). An abdominopelvic mass would indicate a possible pregnancy or hormone-producing ovarian tumour.

A5: What investigations would be most helpful and why?

- **Pregnancy test** ✓ Hospital pregnancy tests are more reliable than home tests.

- **LH and FSH** ✓ An LH:FSH ratio/measurement (taken during menses or just afterwards) of 3:1 was previously taken to indicate PCOS. However, raised LH levels are common, particularly in anovulatory women, and a specific but not very sensitive index of PCOS. Many patients with all of the other clinical and biochemical features of PCOS have normal LH levels. The diagnosis is made primarily on clinical (amenorrhoea/oligomenorrhoea) and ultrasound criteria. The finding of raised testosterone and/or LH merely complements the clinical diagnosis. An FSH level of >25 IU/mL is highly indicative of premature menopause.

- **Serum testosterone** ✓ Serum concentrations of testosterone and other androgens are raised in PCOS, therefore a useful screening test.

- **Serum prolactin** ✓ If hyperprolactinaemia is confirmed, further tests (computed tomography or magnetic resonance imaging of head for pituitary adenoma, and visual field assessment) for prolactinoma may be required.

- **TFT** ✗ This test is required only in cases with symptoms or signs of hypo-/hyperthyroidism, or if there is hyperprolactinaemia, which is known to be associated with hypothyroidism.

- **USS** ± The ultrasound criteria for the diagnosis of a polycystic ovary are eight or more subcapsular follicular cysts <10 mm in diameter and increased ovarian stroma. A thick endometrium is associated with polycystic ovaries, but a thin endometrium is associated with premature menopause.

A6: What treatment options are appropriate?

SUPPORTIVE

- After cessation of excessive training and an increase in body weight, spontaneous resolution and return of menses would be expected.

MEDICAL

- PCOS – combined oral contraceptive (COC) if the patient wishes to have periods. If pregnancy is desired, then commence ovulation induction (see Case 12.2).
- Menopause – COC, combined HRT (see Case 8.3 and OSCE Counselling Case 8.1).
- Hyperprolactinaemia – bromocriptine, cabergoline (dopamine agonists).

SURGERY

- Surgery for pituitary adenoma is rarely required nowadays.
- Ovarian drilling for PCOS.

CASE 8.2 – I have intolerable menstrual periods.

A1: What is the likely differential diagnosis?

- Premenstrual syndrome (PMS).
- Secondary dysmenorrhoea:
  - endometriosis – adenomyosis;
  - pelvic inflammatory disease.
- Pelvic venous congestion.

A2: What issues in the given history support the diagnosis?

Premenstrual syndrome is common around the age of 35 years. This complex problem of unknown aetiology occurs during the week before menstruation and is classically resolved by menstruation. Adenomyosis is associated with painful periods that are usually heavy.

A3: What additional features in the history would you seek to support a particular diagnosis?

Tension, aggression, depression and 'fluid' retention are other common symptoms of PMS. Any susceptibility to accidents, criminal acts and suicide indicates severe disability, which occurs in 3 per cent of cases.

A4: What clinical examination would you perform and why?

General examination with pelvic examination is necessary to exclude 'organic' disease (e.g. pouch of Douglas nodularity, which may be caused by endometriosis). A mental state examination is essential because depression and neurosis can present as PMS.

A5: What investigations would be most helpful and why?

• **Symptom diary**	✓	The diagnosis of PMS is confirmed by establishing that the recurrent symptoms are the same, that they occur regularly and that there is a symptom-free period between menses.
• **USS**	±	A pelvic ultrasound examination may show ovarian endometrioma (termed 'chocolate cysts').
• **Diagnostic laparoscopy**	±	Not required as a routine test, but may be considered if there is any suggestion of an organic cause for the pelvic pain.

A6: What treatment options are appropriate?

SUPPORTIVE

- Treatment is empirical because the cause is unknown. Sympathetic handling, support, reassurance about the absence of pathology and understanding (particularly by family members) are very important.
- Cognitive and relaxation therapy.
- Any treatment has a high (75 per cent) placebo response rate.

MEDICAL

- COC (not progesterone alone).
- Evening primrose oil.
- Vitamin B_6 (pyridoxine).

- Selective serotonin reuptake inhibitors (SSRIs) are effective in severe cases.
- High-dose oestrogens may be helpful, but progestogens would be required as well to prevent endometrial hyperplasia/malignancy.
- Gonadotrophin-releasing hormone agonists can be used to stop ovarian function temporarily. Symptomatic relief is both diagnostic and therapeutic.
- Diuretics are not usually successful.

SURGICAL

- A last-resort permanent solution would be bilateral oophorectomy by performing a concomitant total abdominal hysterectomy. 'Oestrogen-alone' HRT as a non-cyclical preparation may be used subsequently without causing a recurrence of symptoms.

CASE 8.3 – **Should I take HRT?**

A1: What is the likely differential diagnosis?

Menopause.

A2: What issues in the given history support the diagnosis?

The average age of menopause in the UK is 51 years. This patient has had menopausal symptoms for 3 years, indicating that the climacteric and menopause are occurring at the appropriate age.

A3: What additional features in the history would you seek to support a particular diagnosis?

Other symptoms of the menopause include depression, loss of libido, hair loss, dry skin and painful intercourse as a result of a dry vagina (dyspareunia). It is important to check whether there is any family history of osteoporosis, breast cancer or ischaemic heart disease, or early menopause, as well as checking factors such as smoking, previous Colles' or hip fracture, sedentary lifestyle and low body mass index. It would be important to exclude any evidence of vaginal bleeding, which would warrant further investigations (see Case 10.3).

A4: What clinical examination would you perform and why?

General examination, including blood pressure measurement, is necessary to exclude hypertension. Examination of the breasts is mandatory, but it is likely that, if the patient is registered with a general practice, she will have been called for breast screening through the national screening programme initiated at 51 years of age. Pelvic examination would be necessary only if a recent cervical smear had not been taken.

A5: What investigations would be most helpful and why?

The diagnosis of menopause is firm in this case and, therefore, a determination of FSH levels is not required. However, it may be prudent to offer this patient genetic counselling and screening for breast cancer (*BRAC-1* and *BRAC-2* genes) if at least two first-degree relatives (mother or sisters) have had breast cancer.

A6: What treatment options are appropriate?

This patient should be given *combined* oestrogen and progestogen preparations because she has an intact uterus. 'Oestrogen-only' preparations should be prescribed only in patients who have undergone a hysterectomy.

There are several different preparations of HRT available (oral, patches, implants and gel). They can induce monthly withdrawal bleeding, 3-monthly withdrawal bleeding or no withdrawal bleeding. The continuous combined preparations would be highly suitable for this patient because she has been amenorrhoeic for at least a year. This would improve her long-term compliance with HRT.

This patient would need careful counselling about the benefits and disadvantages of HRT because she has a family history of heart disease and breast cancer. Current evidence does not support the use of HRT when there is a history of heart disease and breast cancer, although HRT would not be contraindicated if the patient was adequately counselled (see below). Counselling should be reinforced with written literature.

♔♔ OSCE counselling cases

OSCE COUNSELLING CASE 8.1 – **HRT compliance.**

A1: What issues should be considered for improving this woman's compliance?
- Explore any concerns that she may have about the treatment.
- Ensure that she has realistic expectations of the treatment.
- Emphasize the benefits of treatment – both short-term symptomatic benefits (e.g. relief from flushes) and long-term benefits (e.g. reduced risk of osteoporosis).
- Provide accurate information about the risks and potential complications (e.g. cancer and thromboembolism).
- Discuss the appropriate method of administration and type of HRT for the patient.
- Ensure regular review.
- Give the patient a leaflet/literature about HRT.

A2: What would be an appropriate screening programme for this patient if she were happy to start HRT?
- Pre-treatment:
  - blood pressure measurement;
  - weight;
  - breast examination;
  - cervical smear;
  - pelvic examination.
- Six-monthly:
  - weight;
  - blood pressure measurement.
- Yearly:
  - breast examination.
- Three-yearly:
  - mammography;
  - cervical smear (pelvic examination).

OSCE COUNSELLING CASE 8.2 – **Controversies with HRT.**

A1: What are the benefits and risks of HRT in the light of current evidence?

HRT ADVICE FOR PRESCRIBERS
- For the treatment of menopausal symptoms, the benefits of short-term HRT are considered to outweigh the risks in most women.
- Each decision to start HRT should be made on an individual basis with a fully informed woman.
- In all cases, it is good practice to use the lowest effective dose for the shortest possible time and to review the need to continue treatment at least annually. This review should take into account new knowledge and any changes in a woman's risk factors and personal preferences.
- For postmenopausal women who are at an increased risk of fracture and are aged over 50 years, HRT should be used to prevent osteoporosis only in those who are intolerant of, or contraindicated for, other osteoporosis therapies.

Table 8.1 Benefits and risks associated with using HRT

Condition	Number of cases/1000 non-HRT users	Reduced number of cases in 1000 HRT users over 5 years' HRT use	
		Oestrogen only	Combined HRT
Benefits over 5 years			
Relief of menopausal symptoms, i.e. hot flushes, night sweats, vaginal dryness and discomfort, difficulty in sleeping and consequential depression, mood swings, tiredness and poor concentration		Effective	Effective
Colorectal cancer	6–10	No significant effect	1–3 (± 2)
Fracture of neck of femur	0.5–5.5	0.3–3 (± 2)	0.3–3 (± 2)
Cumulative cancer risk over 5 years		**EXTRA number of cases in 1000 HRT users over 5 years' HRT use**	
Breast cancer	14–16	0–1.5 (± 1.5)	4–6 (± 4)
Endometrial cancer	3	5 (± 1)	Cannot be estimated
Ovarian cancer	3	1 (± 1)	Not known
Cardiovascular risk over 5 years			
Stroke	3–15	2–6 (± 4)	1–4 (± 3)
Venous thromboembolism (VTE)	3–11.5	1–4 (± 4)	4–9 (± 5)
Coronary heart disease (CHD)		No benefit	No benefit
Cognitive function or dementia		No benefit	No benefit

Numbers are best estimates (± approximate range from 95 per cent confidence intervals).

- Women who are receiving HRT for their menopausal symptoms will benefit from the effect of HRT on osteoporosis prevention while on treatment.
- Healthy women who have no menopausal symptoms should be advised against taking HRT because the risks outweigh the benefits.
- HRT does not prevent coronary artery disease or a decline in cognitive function and should not be prescribed for these purposes.
- HRT remains contraindicated in women who have had breast cancer.
- For women without a uterus, oestrogen-only therapy is appropriate.
- For women with a uterus, oestrogen plus progestogen is recommended. However, women should be fully informed of the added risk of breast cancer and be involved in the decision-making process.

A2: How can the HRT preparation be altered to suit her so that she can continue using HRT?

For this patient, the insertion of the levonorgestrel intrauterine system releasing the progestogen component of HRT (with systemic E_2 preparation) may reduce her breast cancer risk because systemic progestogens are implicated in the increase in breast cancer risk. This is extrapolated from the randomized controlled trials data that there is no increase in risk of breast cancer in oestrogen-alone HRT users.

REVISION PANEL

- Weight loss below a certain threshold (e.g. athletes, ballet dancers) or weight gain can cause amenorrhoea.
- PMS is a debilitating condition that requires careful diagnosis, assessment and treatment.
- The modal age of menopause in the UK is 51 years.
- Progestogens as part of HRT are required for endometrial protection, but are implicated in the increased risk of breast cancer.
- Contraception should be continued until 2 years after the last period in women under 50 and 1 year in women over 50 years.

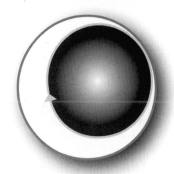

 Incontinence and prolapse

Questions

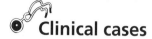

Clinical cases

For each of the case scenarios given, consider the following:

> **Q1**: What is the likely differential diagnosis?
> **Q2**: What issues in the given history support the diagnosis?
> **Q3**: What additional features in the history would you seek to support a particular diagnosis?
> **Q4**: What clinical examination would you perform and why?
> **Q5**: What investigations would be most helpful and why?
> **Q6**: What treatment options are appropriate?

CASE 9.1 – **Every time I cough, I leak urine.**

A 36-year-old parous woman complains of involuntary urinary loss on exercise, sneezing or coughing. She has suffered from this problem since the birth of her first child 10 years earlier, which was assisted with forceps. She is fit and healthy, but has to wear sanitary protection all the time. Otherwise, she voids five or six times a day and once at night, passing good volumes of urine without difficulty.

CASE 9.2 – **I have to rush to the toilet, otherwise I leak urine.**

A 60-year-old woman complains of voiding difficulties. She has frequency of 10–12 times during the day. At night, she gets up three or four times to void. There is also involuntary urinary loss, particularly when she cannot reach the toilet in time. She has had this problem for the last 5 years, but it has gradually been worsening since her periods stopped 10 years ago. She is not on hormone replacement therapy (HRT). Recently, the urinary loss has increased so much that it has become a major hygienic problem. Her social activities have become severely restricted because of the worsening of the condition. She has been treated for urinary tract infections on several occasions in the past. There is no history of diabetes or hypertension.

CASE 9.3 – **I feel something coming down.**

A 56-year-old shopkeeper presents to a gynaecology clinic with a 3-month history of a sensation of 'something coming down'. She feels a 'lump' in her vagina, which is worse towards the end of the day, in association with a dragging backache. She has had four vaginal deliveries, one of which was assisted by forceps. There were no macrosomic babies. She does not have urinary or bowel incontinence.

♟♟ OSCE counselling cases

OSCE COUNSELLING CASE 9.1 – **What investigations am I going to have for leaking urine?**

A 56-year-old woman presents with a history of incontinence of urine and urinary frequency. She describes a sudden urge to pass urine followed by incontinence, but she can also leak when lifting and coughing. You have excluded a urinary tract infection and pelvic examination is unremarkable. You decide to perform urodynamic investigations.

Q1: In counselling this patient, what points would you wish to make about the reasons for performing the investigation?

Q2: What does the investigation involve?

OSCE COUNSELLING CASE 9.2 – **Can my prolapse be treated without surgery?**

A 65-year-old woman is referred with a procidentia that is reducible. There are no pelvic masses or urinary or faecal problems.

Q1: Discuss the non-surgical management options and any potential problems that may be encountered with these treatments, as the patient is medically unfit for surgery.

⟁ Key concepts

In order to work through the core clinical cases in this chapter, you will need to understand the following key concepts.

CONTINENCE

Ability to hold urine in the bladder at all times, except when voiding.

INCONTINENCE

Involuntary urine loss that is objectively demonstrable, which is a social or hygienic problem.

URODYNAMIC STRESS INCONTINENCE (USI)

This was previously called genuine stress incontinence. USI is noted during filling cystometry and is defined as the involuntary leakage of urine during increased abdominal pressure in the absence of a detrusor contraction.

DETRUSOR OVERACTIVITY

This was previously called detrusor instability. Detrusor overactivity is a urodynamic observation characterized by involuntary detrusor contractions during the filling phase, which may be spontaneous or provoked.

FREQUENCY

Normal frequency is usually every 4h. Voiding more often than six times a day or more frequently than every 2h is usually regarded as abnormal.

NOCTURIA

Interruption of sleep as a result of micturition more than once every night. Voiding twice at night over the age of 70 years and three times over the age of 80 years is considered to be within normal limits.

UTEROVAGINAL PROLAPSE

Descent of the pelvic genital organs towards or through the vaginal introitus:
- First degree: descent of the cervix and uterus within the vagina but not up to the introitus.
- Second degree: descent of the cervix and uterus up to the introitus.
- Third degree: descent of the cervix and the whole uterus through the introitus.
- Procidentia: cervix and whole of the uterus completely out of the introitus and is usually accompanied by cystourethrocele and rectocele.

Answers

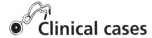 **Clinical cases**

CASE 9.1 – **Every time I cough, I leak urine.**

A1: What is the likely differential diagnosis?

- USI, most likely.
- Detrusor overactivity (urge incontinence).
- Mixed incontinence (USI and detrusor overactivity).
- Neurological disorder (uncommon).

A2: What issues in the given history support the diagnosis?

A history of involuntary urinary loss resulting from a rise in intra-abdominal pressure during exercise, sneezing or coughing in the absence of voiding difficulties is suggestive, but not a definite feature of USI. Difficult childbirth can be a risk factor. Quality of life is measured by the impact of the urinary problem on the patient's usual activities.

A3: What additional features in the history would you seek to support a particular diagnosis?

A specific history of urgency and urge incontinence with or without associated urinary tract infections (UTIs) is suggestive of detrusor overactivity. Urinary frequency is more than five or six times per day, and sleep is also disturbed as a result of nocturnal frequency. Urodynamic stress incontinence will often be associated with multiparity, prolonged labour, and symptoms of uterovaginal prolapse and faecal incontinence. In neurological disorders such as multiple sclerosis, incontinence will usually be a secondary symptom.

A4: What clinical examination would you perform and why?

Physical examination should be performed with a comfortably full bladder, when incontinence should be demonstrated by asking the patient to cough. However, this finding does not conclusively indicate USI. Pelvic examination is usually normal in women with incontinence. Incontinence is sometimes associated with pelvic masses (e.g. a large fibroid uterus causing pressure effects). Occasionally, incontinence is associated with neurological disease. Urodynamic stress incontinence may be associated with evidence of perineal deficiency on inspection and uterovaginal descent on straining.

It is important not to rely solely on the patient's history and examination for diagnosis.

A5: What investigations would be most helpful and why?

- **MSU** ☑ To exclude urinary tract infection.

- **Bladder diary** ☑ To evaluate intake and output with recording episodes of urgency and leakage and precipitating events.

- **Urodynamic investigations** ☑ To differentiate between USI and detrusor overactivity. In USI, urodynamics are normal, i.e.:
  - urine flow rate >15 mL/s (Fig. 9.1);
  - bladder capacity >300 mL;
  - residual volume <50 mL;
  - bladder pressure rises by <15 cm H$_2$O during filling;
  - detrusor remains stable throughout filling and voiding.

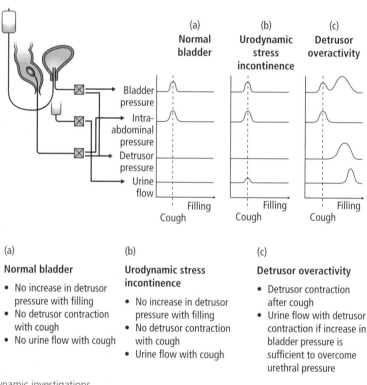

(a) **Normal bladder**
- No increase in detrusor pressure with filling
- No detrusor contraction with cough
- No urine flow with cough

(b) **Urodynamic stress incontinence**
- No increase in detrusor pressure with filling
- No detrusor contraction with cough
- Urine flow with cough

(c) **Detrusor overactivity**
- Detrusor contraction after cough
- Urine flow with detrusor contraction if increase in bladder pressure is sufficient to overcome urethral pressure

Figure 9.1 Urodynamic investigations.

A6: What treatment options are appropriate?

SUPPORTIVE

The local incontinence advisory service should be involved in management. USI can be treated conservatively using techniques for pelvic floor re-education (pelvic floor exercises and other physiotherapy techniques, including vaginal cones, perineometry, electrical stimulation).

MEDICAL

- Drug therapy includes α-agonists (e.g. phenylpropanolamine), which increase urethral resistance.

SURGICAL

- Surgery is used to support the proximal urethra and to elevate the bladder neck to restore the suburethral hammock support. This is commonly done using retropubic and transobturator tapes (tension-free tapes) and previously colposuspension. Alternative surgical techniques include paraurethral bulking. These techniques should be employed in preference to anterior colporrhaphy and anterior repair, which do not have the desired long-term benefits compared with colposuspension procedures.

CASE 9.2 – I have to rush to the toilet, otherwise I leak urine.

A1: What is the likely differential diagnosis?

- Detrusor overactivity (urge incontinence), most likely.
- Urodynamic stress incontinence.
- Mixed incontinence (USI and detrusor overactivity).
- Neurological disorder (uncommon).

A2: What issues in the given history support the diagnosis?

A history of urgency, frequency and nocturia with or without associated UTIs is highly suggestive of detrusor overactivity. At this patient's age, frequency every 2 h is abnormal. Quality of life is measured by the patient's social activities being restricted and her having hygiene problems. Postmenopausal atrophic changes of the bladder will also be a contributory factor in this case.

A3: What additional features in the history would you seek to support a particular diagnosis?

Fluid intake habits, particularly in relation to tea, coffee and alcohol, are important with regard to the symptomatology. Haematuria may indicate a bladder stone or tumour. Involuntary urine loss as a result of a rise in intra-abdominal pressure (e.g. caused by exercise, sneezing or coughing) in the absence of voiding difficulties is suggestive of USI. Incontinence may be associated with symptoms of uterovaginal prolapse and faecal incontinence. In neurological disorders such as multiple sclerosis, incontinence will usually be a secondary symptom.

A4: What clinical examination would you perform and why?

Physical examination should be performed with a comfortably full bladder, when incontinence may be demonstrated by asking the patient to cough. Signs of oestrogen deficiency may be evident on inspection of the genitalia. There may be uterovaginal descent on straining. Pelvic examination may reveal a pelvic mass, which may be the cause of urinary symptoms resulting from pressure effects. Occasionally, incontinence is associated with neurological disease. Examination of S2, S3 and S4 dermatomes is essential.

A5: What investigations would be most helpful and why?

- **MSU** ✓   To exclude urinary tract infection.

- **Bladder diary** ✓

- **Urodynamic investigations** ☑ To differentiate between USI and detrusor overactivity. In detrusor overactivity, urodynamics might show:
  - reduced bladder capacity (<300 mL);
  - high bladder pressure, increasing to >15 cm H_2O during filling;
  - spontaneous detrusor contractions during filling, or contractions in response to provocation such as a change in posture.

  Urodynamic investigations are not essential as a matter of routine. They should, however, be undertaken in patients who are not responding to supportive and medical therapeutic measures.

- **Cystoscopy** ☑ In resistant cases.

A6: What treatment options are appropriate?

SUPPORTIVE

The incontinence advisory service should be involved in management. Fluid intake habits may have to be altered in order to manage the symptoms (e.g. last drink at 18:00, reducing tea, coffee and alcohol intake). Detrusor overactivity can be treated conservatively using techniques for bladder training and bladder drill to re-establish central bladder control.

MEDICAL

Drug therapy in this case might include HRT. Urinary tract infections should be treated with appropriate antibiotics. Anticholinergic drugs include oxybutynin, tolterodine and newer drugs include solifenacin, fesoterodine and darifenacin. Side effects include dry mouth, blurred vision and constipation.

SURGICAL

There is no place for surgery as a primary intervention. Only when all other methods have been exhausted should complex procedures such as clam cystoplasty be considered. These are end-stage procedures with a high morbidity rate and long-term problems.

CASE 9.3 – I feel something coming down.

A1: What is the likely differential diagnosis?

- Cystocele.
- Uterine prolapse:
  - first degree;
  - second degree;
  - third degree (procidentia).
- Rectocele.
- (Enterocele – pouch of Douglas hernia, which contains loops of bowel.)

A2: What issues in the given history support the diagnosis?

'Something coming down' is a symptom of the various types of uterovaginal prolapse (Fig. 9.2). Prolapse premenopausally is uncommon. Childbirth and particularly traumatic delivery indicates that there may have been possible pelvic floor damage. It is difficult to ascertain the type of prolapse from the history

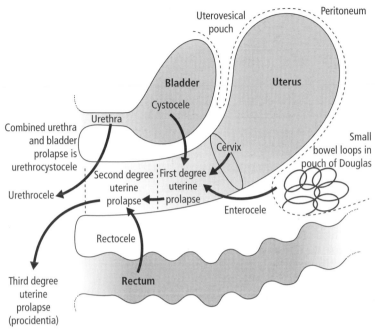

Peritoneum

Uterovesical
pouch

Bladder **Uterus**

Cystocele

Urethra

Combined urethra
and bladder
prolapse is
urethrocystocele

Cérvix

Small
bowel loops in
pouch of Douglas

Second degree First degree
uterine   uterine
prolapse   prolapse

Urethrocele

Enterocele

Rectocele

Rectum

Third degree
uterine
prolapse
(procidentia)

Figure 9.2 Different types of prolapse.

alone without examination. It is said that women who have a physically demanding job are at high risk of prolapse. The sensation of prolapse is typically worse at the end of the day.

A3: What additional features in the history would you seek to support a particular diagnosis?

It is important to ascertain a history of urinary incontinence (see Cases 9.1 and 9.2). In general, stress incontinence is not associated with cystocele. Constipation or difficulty on emptying fully can suggest a rectocele. The use of HRT may reduce the risk of prolapse. Postnatal exercises are considered to be a preventive measure for future prolapse. Smoking history and cough associated with respiratory illnesses may exacerbate the symptoms of prolapse. Chronic cough is a poor prognostic factor for the success of prolapse surgery. It is also important to establish whether the patient is sexually active as any potential surgery can affect sexual function (see A6 below).

A4: What clinical examination would you perform and why?

Record the patient's weight and perform a general physical examination to assess her fitness for surgery, if this is intended. Exclude an abdominal mass and examine the external genitalia to assess signs of atrophy. Ask the patient to cough in order to detect any stress incontinence (although elicitation of this at the time of examination is not conclusive evidence of her incontinence). During straining, any components of prolapse can be described, but the different types can be distinguished only using a Sim's speculum in the left lateral position. A bimanual examination should be performed to exclude a pelvic mass.

A5: What investigations would be most helpful and why?

The diagnosis is primarily made on the basis of the clinical examination. If there is concurrent incontinence, urodynamics would be mandatory before surgery (see OSCE Counselling Case 9.1).

A6: What treatment options are appropriate?

SUPPORTIVE

- Weight control.
- To stop smoking.
- Pelvic floor exercises.
- Vaginal pessaries (e.g. ring or shelf) may be used to provide symptom relief if the patient is unfit for surgery or wishes to avoid surgery. Pessaries are more likely to be helpful in women with a prominent suprapubic arch and strong perineal body for support; otherwise, the pessary is easily expelled. Pessaries are generally replaced every 6 months.

MEDICAL

Vaginal oestrogen cream or HRT.

SURGICAL

- Cystocele: anterior repair (colporrhaphy).
- Uterovaginal prolapse: cervical amputation with shortening of the uterosacral ligaments (Manchester–Fothergill repair). This operation should be performed only if a vaginal hysterectomy is not possible.
- Vaginal hysterectomy: this removes the prolapsed organ. Anterior repair and posterior repair are performed if appropriate. The vaginal vault should be suspended.
- Rectocele: posterior repair and perineal repair in cases where there is a deficient perineum from previous childbirth (posterior colpoperineorrhaphy).

In all surgical interventions, the rate of recurrence is high if preventive measures are not implemented (e.g. using HRT, reduction in body weight and stopping smoking in the case of chronic cough). In any repair operation, the vagina and introitus should not be obliterated, which would inhibit intercourse and possibly be a cause of dyspareunia.

👥 OSCE counselling cases

OSCE COUNSELLING CASE 9.1 – **What investigations am I going to have for leaking urine?**

A1: In counselling this patient, what points would you wish to make about the reasons for performing the investigation?

- Urodynamics measures the pressure in the bladder and how the bladder works when it is filled and emptied.
- The performance of the test will identify why the woman's incontinence is occurring (i.e. whether it is caused by a weakness in the supports of the bladder neck, or whether it occurs because the bladder is sensitive and contracts with even little urine in it).
- It is important to differentiate between USI and detrusor overactivity, because the treatment for each problem is different, i.e. surgical options for USI and medical options for detrusor overactivity. Using the surgical option for detrusor overactivity could make the patient's problem worse.
- The procedure is performed in the outpatient clinic without any analgesia or anaesthesia.

A2: What does the investigation involve?

- A catheter is placed in the patient's bladder and in her back passage (rectum).
- Some minor discomfort may be experienced when the catheters are inserted.
- Each is connected to a machine that measures bladder and abdominal pressure.
- The bladder is filled through the catheter in the bladder, and the pressure in the bladder is measured while this is being done. The amount of fluid present in the patient's bladder before she feels that she needs to pass water will be measured.
- She will then be asked to stand up and cough, to see whether urine leaks.
- Finally, she will be asked to empty her bladder into the commode so that the flow rate can be measured.
- The patient will be followed up in the clinic after the results of the test have been obtained.

OSCE COUNSELLING CASE 9.2 – **Can my prolapse be treated without surgery?**

A1: Discuss the non-surgical management options and any potential problems that may be encountered with these treatments, as the patient is medically unfit for surgery.

MANAGEMENT OPTIONS

- No treatment and just reassurance if the patient remains problem free. The procidentia is unlikely to cause any serious harm, but it is considered to be a progressive condition.
- Topical weekly/twice weekly oestrogen application in the vagina to counteract excoriation and dryness. Alternatively, combined HRT can be prescribed.
- To help to keep the procidentia reduced, insert a ring pessary of appropriate size.
- If the ring pessary fails to stay in place, a shelf pessary of appropriate size should be tried. This has a higher likelihood of success, but is usually incompatible with sexual function.

PROBLEMS

- Ring and shelf pessaries will require replacement every 6 months. They can cause bleeding as a result of pressure on atrophic vaginal skin. If excoriation or ulceration occurs, the pessaries should be left out and topical oestrogen cream prescribed daily for 2–4 weeks. Reinsertion is appropriate after complete healing.
- Sometimes the pessaries can cause urinary retention and/or faecal impaction.

REVISION PANEL

- Urinary incontinence has a high prevalence, affecting approximately 20–30 per cent of the adult female population.
- The most common causes of urinary incontinence are USI and detrusor overactivity.
- The mainstays of treatment for USI are physiotherapy and surgery, whereas for detrusor overactivity, these are bladder retraining and anticholinergic medication.
- Childbirth injury is the major aetiological factor in organ prolapse.

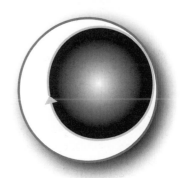

10 Neoplasia

Questions

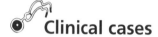 **Clinical cases**

For each of the case scenarios given, consider the following:

Q1: What is the likely differential diagnosis?
Q2: What issues in the given history support the diagnosis?
Q3: What additional features in the history would you seek to support a particular diagnosis?
Q4: What clinical examination would you perform and why?
Q5: What investigations would be most helpful and why?
Q6: What treatment options are appropriate?

CASE 10.1 – **My cervical screening test is abnormal.**

A 35-year-old single woman is found to have an abnormal test on routine screening. She has had regular tests since the age of 25 years, and previous results have been normal. She has two children aged 2 and 7 years. She is separated from her partner, who fathered both children. She is currently using the oral contraceptive pill; she is not in a stable relationship.

CASE 10.2 – **I am menopausal and my abdomen is distending.**

A 68-year-old woman presents with gradual enlargement of the abdomen, changes in bowel habit and weight loss. The general practitioner had felt a lower abdominal mass and referred the patient urgently to the gynaecology clinic.

CASE 10.3 – **I have gone through the change and I have recently had some vaginal bleeding.**

A 54-year-old woman has been amenorrhoeic for the past 18 months, and recently had an episode of fresh vaginal bleeding. Her last cervical screening test, taken 2 years ago, was normal. She is not on hormone replacement therapy (HRT).

⚥ OSCE counselling cases

OSCE COUNSELLING CASE 10.1 – **My cervical screening test report is abnormal. Do I have cancer?**

Having had a routine cervical screening test 2 weeks earlier, a 36-year-old woman returns to see you (her GP) about the result. She has received a card through the post indicating that the test has shown an abnormailty and she is very anxious about the implications of this.

The test result, which you have available, is as follows:
- Good cellularity.
- Endocervical cells present.
- Moderate dyskaryosis.

Q1: Counsel this patient about her screening test result.

OSCE COUNSELLING CASE 10.2 – **I have warts. Will I get cancer?**

A 26-year-old woman presents with genital warts. She is worried that the virus that causes warts also causes cervical cancer. She has never had a cervical screening test.

Q1: What would you say to her?

Key concepts

In order to work through the core clinical cases in this chapter, you will need to understand the following key concepts.

- Human papillomavirus (HPV) infection leads to premalignant change in the cervical epithelium, to result in cervical intraepithelial neoplasia (CIN), which has the potential to turn malignant.
- There are over 100 different virus types of HPV, with types 6 and 11 causing genital warts, and types 16, 18, 31 and 33 having oncogenic cancer properties.
- The National Health Service Cervical Screening Programme (NHSCSP) in the UK tests women aged between 25 and 49 years every 3 years, and women aged between 50 and 64 years every 5 years.
- In the UK, the 'Pap' smear has been superseded by liquid-based cytology (LBC), in which a small brush is used to sample cells from the transformation zone and the cells examined cytologically to indicate different degrees of maturity (dyskaryosis – borderline, mild, moderate and severe).
- LBC has reduced the number of inadequate samples from over 9 per cent before LBC to 2.5 per cent.
- Only histological analysis of cervical tissue can give a definitive diagnosis of CIN.
- In the UK, a national programme of HPV vaccination for girls aged 12–13 and 17–18 years started in 2009 to prevent HPV types 16 and 18 (types found in over 99 per cent of cervical cancers).

Answers

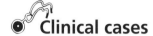

Clinical cases

CASE 10.1 – **My cervical screening test is abnormal.**

A1: What is the likely differential diagnosis?

An abnormal screening test could be associated with:
- Infection or inflammation.
- Dyskaryosis (which may be reflective of cervical intraepithelial neoplasia) (see Fig. 10.1).
- Malignancy.

A2: What issues in the given history support the diagnosis?

Although an abnormal screening test often leads to concern about cancer, in most cases, it is associated with a benign condition (infection, inflammation or cervical intraepithelial neoplasia). From the given history, one can elicit only some of the risk factors for cervical intraepithelial neoplasia (e.g. multiparity and multiple sexual partners). However, it is not possible to be certain of the diagnosis without further investigation.

A3: What additional features in the history would you seek to support a particular diagnosis?

The history of additional risk factors associated with cervical intraepithelial neoplasia and cancer should be obtained, e.g. young age at first intercourse, sexually transmitted infection, particularly HPV and herpes simplex virus 2 (HSV-2), cigarette smoking and low socioeconomic status. Gynaecological symptoms such as intermenstrual bleeding and postcoital bleeding may be indicative of a local lesion. Vaginal discharge may be associated with infection or inflammation. The current partner's history of sexually transmitted infection may be relevant.

A4: What clinical examination would you perform and why?

Inspection of the vulva and vagina may reveal discharge or infection. Inspection of the cervix may show a cervical ectropion, a polyp or a tumour. In most cases, however, cervical inspection with the naked eye will be normal. Bimanual examination should be performed to assess for a cervical mass, cervical fixity, pelvic mass and pelvic tenderness. In the case of cervical cancer, examination will also determine staging, but this is usually performed under anaesthesia together with cystoscopy. If a sexually transmitted infection is diagnosed, the male partner will also need to be examined and tested.

A5: What investigations would be most helpful and why?

- **Colposcopy and cervical biopsies** ☑ If the abnormality in the screening test shows moderate or severe dyskaryosis, colposcopy (inspection of the cervix under magnification using a binocular microscope) should be performed. During colposcopy, directed biopsy samples should be taken to establish a histological diagnosis.

- **Cervical and vaginal swabs** ± If infection is suspected, appropriate vaginal and cervical swabs should be obtained for microbiological investigation.

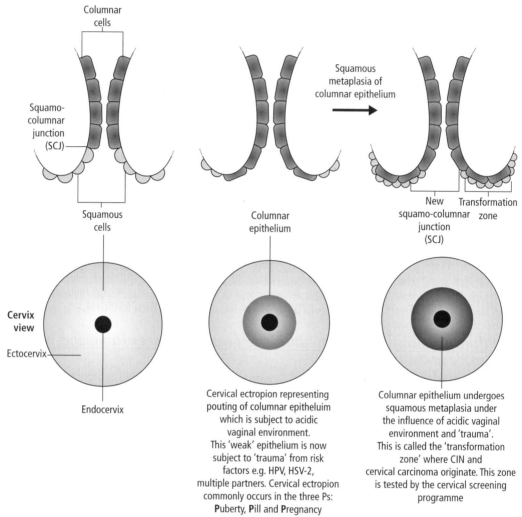

Figure 10.1 Mechanisms of abnormal cervical screening tests. HPV, human papillomavirus; HSV, herpes simplex virus; CIN, cervical intraepithelial neoplasia.

A6: What treatment options are appropriate?

SUPPORTIVE

Explanation depending on findings of clinical examination and degree of abnormality of screening test report and need for further investigation and follow-up. The specific treatment depends on the cause.

MEDICAL

Infection: treat according to cause and repeat the test after 6 months.

SURGICAL

- Cervical ectropion: observation only, or cryotherapy for symptomatic relief for troublesome postcoital bleeding.
- Cervical intraepithelial neoplasia: excision or ablation of the lesion and follow-up tests.

- Cervical cancer: chest radiograph, intravenous urogram, cystoscopy, examination under anaesthetic, cervical biopsy, surgery and/or radiotherapy according to stage.

Table 10.1 Appropriate actions to be taken in response to cervical screening test report

Cervical screening test report	Appropriate action
Normal	Repeat test every 3 or 5 years depending on age
Inadequate	Repeat
Borderline	Repeat test at 6 months – if abnormality is persistent, refer for colposcopy
Mild dyskaryosis	Refer for colposcopy or repeat test after no more than 6 months. If abnormality persists, refer for colposcopy
Moderate/severe dyskaryosis	Refer for colposcopy
Suspected invasive cancer or glandular abnormalities	Refer urgently to colposcopy for cone biopsy, hysteroscopy

CASE 10.2 – I am menopausal and my abdomen is distending.

A1: What is the likely differential diagnosis?
- Pelvic mass arising from the ovary, fallopian tube or uterus.
- Ascites.
- Bladder distension.
- Bowel problems (e.g. flatus, faeces, cancer).

A2: What issues in the given history support the diagnosis?
Gradual abdominal distension and changes in bowel habits in a postmenopausal patient with a pelvic mass are highly suspicious of an ovarian tumour.

A3: What additional features in the history would you seek to support a particular diagnosis?
Nulliparity, early menarche, late menopause, higher social class and history of breast cancer are associated with ovarian neoplasm. Use of the oral contraceptive pill has a protective effect. Postmenopausal bleeding can be a symptom of ovarian cancer, but it may also be the result of endometrial or fallopian tube cancer. A urinary and bowel history should be obtained. The diagnosis cannot be definitively established without further investigation.

A4: What clinical examination would you perform and why?
A general examination should be performed, looking for lymphadenopathy and lower limb oedema. Chest examination should specifically exclude pleural effusion. Ascites should be elicited on abdominal examination. Ascites is dull to percussion in the flanks, compared with central dullness in an ovarian cyst. Bimanual examination will detect pelvic mass and delineate the mobility and relationship to the uterus.

A5: What investigations would be most helpful and why?

Investigations should be performed to exclude ovarian tumour.

- CA-125   ☑   This is an ovarian tumour marker.

- USS   ☑   Abdominopelvic ultrasound examination can demonstrate the presence of ascites. If a mass is detected, its nature (whether cystic or solid) and origin may be determined by the scan.

- Chest radiograph   ☑   This may be required in order to assess pleural effusion, or as a preoperative test for fitness for anaesthesia.

- Ascitic sample   ±   This may be taken for cytological examination.

- MRI   ±   If USS is not helpful.

A6: What treatment options are appropriate?

SUPPORTIVE

- Pain relief and drainage of ascites or pleural effusions.

SURGICAL

- Surgical excision of tumour (hysterectomy, bilateral salpingo-oophorectomy, omentectomy and debulking of tumour, aiming to reduce the tumour bulk to <2 cm in diameter).

MEDICAL

- Chemotherapy, depending on the stage determined at surgery.

CASE 10.3 – I have gone through the change and I have recently had some vaginal bleeding.

A1: What is the likely differential diagnosis?

- Atrophic vaginitis.
- Endometrial polyp, hyperplasia and carcinoma.
- Cervical polyp and cancer.
- Adnexal malignancy (uncommon).

A2: What issues in the given history support the diagnosis?

This vaginal bleeding is classified as postmenopausal bleeding (PMB), with a 10–15 per cent likelihood of endometrial pathology, particularly endometrial cancer. Further investigations are therefore mandatory to exclude this.

A3: What additional features in the history would you seek to support a particular diagnosis?

Postcoital bleeding could also suggest a cervical polyp or cancer. Hypertension, diabetes and obesity are risk factors for endometrial hyperplasia and cancer. Information about cervical screening reports must be obtained, bearing in mind that a negative screening history does not exclude the possibility of cervical cancer in women with symptoms of postmenopausal bleeding. Symptoms of hot flushes and night sweats may indicate that any HRT dose taken may not have been sufficient. In this case, there might also be a history of painful dry vagina during intercourse, which would suggest atrophic vaginitis.

A4: What clinical examination would you perform and why?

A general examination should be performed to exclude pallor and lymphadenopathy. Speculum examination will exclude local causes such as atrophic vaginitis and cervical polyps or cervical carcinoma. Bimanual examination should be performed to assess uterine size, mobility and adnexal pathology.

A5: What investigations would be most helpful and why?

The primary aim of investigations is to exclude gynaecological cancer, particularly endometrial cancer.

• **USS**	✓	A pelvic ultrasound examination is performed for endometrial thickness measurement and adnexal masses (ovarian tumours can present as PMB). Current evidence suggests that a regular, thin endometric and an endometrial thickness (ET) of <4 mm substantially reduces the likelihood of endometrial cancer. Endometrial biopsy would then not be required unless there were additional USS features of endometrial irregularity and fluid.
• **Outpatient endometrial biopsy**	✓	It is mandatory to obtain an endometrial sample for histological assessment if the endometrial thickness is ≥ 4 mm.
• **Outpatient hysteroscopy**	±	Only required if there is a failure to get an endometrial biopsy in the outpatient setting or biopsy results are reported as insufficient with an ET ≥ 4 mm, or if an endometrial polyp is suspected on USS. This allows direct visualization of the uterine cavity, which is particularly useful for excluding endometrial polyps.
• **Inpatient D&C**	±	Only required if outpatient assessment is impossible to perform.

A6: What treatment options are appropriate?

SUPPORTIVE

No pathology is found in most cases. If this is so after thorough investigations, then the patient can be reassured.

MEDICAL

- Vaginal oestrogen cream would supplement the existing HRT for treatment of atrophic vaginitis. Alternatively, the HRT dose may be altered to provide a preparation with higher oestrogen content.
- Progestogens (oral/LNG-IUS) for endometrial hyperplasia without atypia. Follow-up biopsies would be required to ensure regression.

SURGICAL

- Polypectomy.
- For complex endometrial hyperplasia with associated atypia, total hysterectomy and bilateral salpingo-oophorectomy would be mandatory as the risk of progression to endometrial cancer can be as high as 40 per cent in untreated cases.
- If endometrial cancer or another gynaecological cancer is detected, it is treated according to stage.

ᴬᴬ OSCE counselling cases

OSCE COUNSELLING CASE 10.1 – **My cervical screening test report is abnormal. Do I have cancer?**

A1: Counsel this patient about her screening test result.

The nature of the report:
- Does not indicate cancer.
- Indicates that abnormal cells are present.
- Requires further investigation to exclude pathology; the pathology is usually a precancerous condition.
- Suggests that, if a precancerous condition is found, it will require further treatment to prevent progression.

The nature of the investigation and treatment would be as follows:
- Referral for colposcopy (examination of the cervix with magnifying binoculars).
- The need for punch biopsies or large loop excision of the transformation zone (LLETZ).
- Treatment by laser/cold coagulation/LLETZ.

Regular follow-up screening tests would be needed according to the findings.

OSCE COUNSELLING CASE 10.2 – **I have warts. Will I get cancer?**

A1: What would you say to her?

- Many factors are associated with the development of cervical cancer and the virus that causes warts is just one of them.
- The wart virus is very common and there are many different types. Not all of these types are associated with cervical cancer.
- Even if the warts are caused by a type of virus that is associated with cervical cancer, the risk of developing it is small.
- Regular cervical screening tests will identify cervical change before the development of cervical cancer. These changes are easily cured before they become cancerous.
- Perform a speculum examination (to confirm that the cervix appears normal) and take a cervical screening test. One should be taken every 3 years.

REVISION PANEL

- In the UK, the National Health Service Cervical Screening Programme has prevented up to 70 per cent of cervical cancer deaths since its inception in 1988.
- Other HPV types have been implicated in the pathogenesis of cervical cancer and the long-term benefits of the HPV types vaccine remain unknown.
- There is some correlation between cervical screening test grade, i.e. low (borderline and mild) or high (moderate and severe) grade dyskaryosis and the degrees of CIN I, II, III, but it is not totally reliable.
- Most investigations for PMB are now carried out in the outpatient setting, using local anaesthesia for difficult cases only.

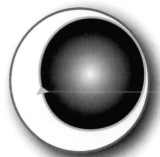

11 Discharge and pain

Questions

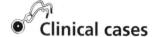

Clinical cases

For each of the case scenarios given, consider the following:

> **Q1**: What is the likely differential diagnosis?
> **Q2**: What issues in the given history support the diagnosis?
> **Q3**: What additional features in the history would you seek to support a particular diagnosis?
> **Q4**: What clinical examination would you perform and why?
> **Q5**: What investigations would be most helpful and why?
> **Q6**: What treatment options are appropriate?

CASE 11.1 – I have constant irritating vaginal discharge.

A 25-year-old single woman has vulval and vaginal itching and discharge. Her recent cervical smear was normal. She has recently started a new relationship and is currently using the oral contraceptive pill. There are no urinary symptoms. She recently had a severe bout of flu for which she was given antibiotics.

CASE 11.2 – I am unwell and have abdominal pain and discharge.

A 22-year-old woman presents with fever, lower abdominal and pelvic pain, and a foul-smelling vaginal discharge. Her last menstrual period was 1 week ago. She has recently changed her sexual partner. There are no urinary or bowel symptoms.

CASE 11.3 – My periods are painful and I also have pain during intercourse.

A 30-year-old nulliparous professional woman presents with severe and incapacitating menstrual pain that requires bed-rest and interferes with her employment. The menstrual pain has been present for 1 year, but it has gradually been increasing in severity over the last few months. The patient's periods are not heavy and she has no desire for fertility. She recently started a relationship and finds intercourse painful. The couple have been using condoms for contraception.

ii OSCE counselling cases

OSCE COUNSELLING CASE 11.1 – I am having a diagnostic laparoscopy. Should I be concerned?

A patient with chronic pelvic pain is going to be admitted to hospital for diagnostic laparoscopy under general anaesthesia. Her clinical pelvic examination and ultrasound scan (USS) are normal.

Q1: What information will you need to provide when counselling her about the investigation?

OSCE COUNSELLING CASE 11.2 – I have had a diagnostic laparoscopy. What happens next?

The above patient underwent an uneventful diagnostic laparoscopy. The laparoscopic findings are of a normal pelvis.

Q1: What information will you need to provide when counselling her before discharge from hospital?

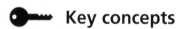

🔑 Key concepts

In order to work through the core clinical cases in this chapter, you will need to understand the following key concepts.

PELVIC INFLAMMATORY DISEASE

Infection of the upper genital tract, with salpingitis as the most prominent feature:
- Primary PID: caused by infection ascending from the lower genital tract.
- Secondary PID: caused by direct spread from adjacent organs, e.g. appendix.

SEXUALLY TRANSMITTED INFECTION

Genital tract infection caused by sexually transmitted infective organisms (e.g. gonorrhoea, *Chlamydia* sp., herpes). Pelvic inflammatory disease is a serious complication of a sexually transmitted infection (STI).

CHRONIC PELVIC PAIN

Constant or intermittent, cyclic or acyclic pain located in the pelvis, which may or may not be related to menstruation, is associated with adverse effects on quality of life and has lasted for more than 6 months. No pelvic pathology is found in 50–60 per cent of cases with chronic pelvic pain.

DYSMENORRHOEA

Pain associated with menstruation:
- Primary dysmenorrhoea: pain not associated with any organic disease. It is common at menarche.
- Secondary dysmenorrhoea: pain associated with organic disease such as endometriosis or PID.

DYSPAREUNIA

Pain associated with sexual intercourse. This can be classified as superficial or deep.

Answers

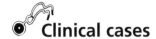 **Clinical cases**

CASE 11.1 – I have constant irritating vaginal discharge.

A1: What is the likely differential diagnosis?

- Infection:
  - *Candida* sp. (thrush);
  - *Trichomonas vaginalis*;
  - bacterial vaginosis;
  - *Chlamydia* sp.;
  - gonorrhoea;
  - herpes.
- Inflammation.
- Foreign body, e.g. forgotten tampon.
- No pathology, e.g. cervical ectropion.

A2: What issues in the given history support the diagnosis?

Associated itching, a new sexual partner, use of the oral contraceptive pill and recent use of broad-spectrum antibiotics could all be associated with candida infection (although most infections involve a mixture of organisms). Urinary symptoms, absent in this case, could be associated with chlamydial infection, gonorrhoea or herpes.

A3: What additional features in the history would you seek to support a particular diagnosis?

Specific enquiry should be directed towards the colour and consistency of the discharge. Typically, a thick white discharge is caused by *Candida* sp., a thin green discharge is associated with bacterial vaginosis, a grey frothy discharge results from *Trichomonas* sp., and a yellow mucopurulent discharge is caused by *Chlamydia* or gonococci. The relationship between discharge and menstruation should be established. Candida infection is usually premenstrual and gonococcal infection is postmenstrual. Intense itching that is worse at night is a feature of candidiasis, but could be associated with trichomonas infection. Pain, dyspareunia and burning are features of trichomonas and gonococcal infections. Poor personal hygiene and use of talcum powder, deodorants, douches and tight synthetic undergarments may lead to itching. The history of an STI in the woman's partner should also be obtained. A family history of diabetes and symptoms of polyuria and polydipsia may indicate diabetes mellitus, which is associated with candida infections.

A4: What clinical examination would you perform and why?

Inspection of the vulva may reveal erythema or congestion, which is much more marked with candida than with trichomonas infection. The erythema may extend perianally. Gonococcal infection may be associated with painful vulval swelling and urethral discharge. Multiple small vesicles with ulcers are associated with herpes. Speculum examination may demonstrate discharge with associated erythema. Trichomonas infection is associated with reddish–purple spots in the vagina and cervix (strawberry cervix). A search should be made for any foreign bodies, e.g. a forgotten tampon. A sample of the discharge should be taken for microscopy, culture and sensitivity. Cervical ectropion may be a cause of discharge without infection. A bimanual examination should be performed to assess pelvic tenderness, which may suggest PID. The male partner should also be examined and tested.

A5: What investigations would be most helpful and why?

- **Urine dipstick** ☑ For glycosuria, leucocytes and nitrites.

- **MSU** ☑ For microscopy and culture.

- **pH of discharge** ☑ The pH of the discharge is more alkaline (>5) in trichomonas infections or bacterial vaginosis. Normal vaginal pH is an acidic environment of 3.5–4.5.

- **Whiff test of discharge** ☑ If the discharge is mixed with potassium hydroxide, it produces a fishy odour in bacterial vaginosis.

- **Microscopy of discharge** ☑ A sample of the discharge should be mixed with saline and examined under the microscope. No organisms are usually seen in physiological discharge. Mycelial filaments and spores are seen in candida infection. Motile flagellated protozoa may be seen in trichomonas infection.

- **Gram stain of discharge** ☑ Gram staining of the discharge will show blue cells with a serrated border in bacterial vaginosis, and Gram-negative diplococci in gonococcal infection.

- **Vaginal and cervical swabs** ☑ Depending on the patient's risk factors for STIs and the findings at examination, swabs should be obtained from the upper vagina, endocervix and urethra for culture. Separate swabs should be taken for *Chlamydia* sp. Investigations of the male partner should also be carried out.

A6: What treatment options are appropriate?

SUPPORTIVE

Advice on personal hygiene and clothing. Specific treatment depends on the cause.

MEDICAL

- No organisms – no treatment if the problem is not persistent. Otherwise, treat as candida infection.
- *Candida* – clotrimazole cream or oral fluconazole.
- *Trichomonas* or bacterial vaginosis – metronidazole.
- *Chlamydia* – doxycycline, azithromycin single dose.
- Gonococci – penicillin, erythromycin.
- Herpes – aciclovir.
- Treat the male partner simultaneously.

SURGICAL

Cervical ectropion – observation only, or cryotherapy for symptomatic relief.

CASE 11.2 – I am unwell and have abdominal pain and discharge.

A1: What is the likely differential diagnosis?

- Acute PID:
  - STI;
  - iatrogenic cause (e.g. caused by intrauterine contraceptive device);
  - secondary PID.
- Acute abdomen:
  - ectopic pregnancy;
  - ovarian cyst/torsion;
  - conditions related to bowel, e.g. irritable bowel syndrome/constipation.

A2: What issues in the given history support the diagnosis?

Pyrexia, pelvic pain and foul-smelling vaginal discharge are probably the result of PID. A recent change of sexual partner is a risk factor for PID. Although ectopic pregnancy is unlikely because this patient's last menstrual period was 1 week ago, ectopic pregnancy should be considered because menstrual history is an unreliable indicator of pregnancy.

A3: What additional features in the history would you seek to support a particular diagnosis?

Specific enquiry should be directed towards the nature and onset of the pain and the pattern of fever. Swinging high-grade pyrexia is typically associated with a pelvic abscess. A sexual history should be obtained, enquiring about the number of sexual partners, any recent casual sexual encounters, history of STIs and previous history of PID. The oral contraceptive pill reduces the risk of PID, but does not necessarily prevent it. Copper intrauterine contraceptive devices, recent gynaecological surgery, delivery or miscarriage are associated with PID.

A4: What clinical examination would you perform and why?

General examination should include measurement of temperature, blood pressure and pulse to assess shock. Inspection of the vulva, vagina and cervix may demonstrate discharge with associated erythema. A sample of the discharge should be taken for microbiology. Separate swabs for gonococci and *Chlamydia* sp. should be taken from the endocervix and urethra. Digital examination of the cervix may elicit excitation. Bimanual examination should be performed to assess pelvic tenderness, which may suggest PID. It may also reveal a mass, e.g. pelvic abscess/ovarian cyst.

A5: What investigations would be most helpful and why?

Investigation		Reason
Urine hCG	✓	To exclude pregnancy.
FBC	✓	A full blood count (FBC) should be taken for leucocytosis.
U&Es	✓	If sepsis is suspected.
USS	✓	A pelvic ultrasound examination should be performed to support clinical examination, particularly excluding any pelvic masses, e.g. pelvic abscess/ovarian cyst.
MSU	✓	For microscopy and culture.
Vaginal and cervical swabs	✓	Samples of the discharge should be examined under the microscope, with Gram staining and culture.
Blood cultures	±	Only if there are signs of septicaemia.

A6: What treatment options are appropriate?

SUPPORTIVE

If there is clinical shock, resuscitation should be performed while examination and investigations are being undertaken. An indwelling catheter should be used to monitor urine output.

MEDICAL

Oxygen, fluid resuscitation and intravenous broad-spectrum antibiotics should be administered in cases of septic shock. Otherwise, treat PID with antibiotics according to the suspected organism or culture and sensitivity reports.

SURGICAL

Once the patient is relatively stable, surgery may be required, depending on the diagnosis:
- PID with pelvic mass that is not responding to medical treatment requires surgical drainage of abscess.
- Acute abdomen – laparotomy.

CASE 11.3 – **My periods are painful and I also have pain during intercourse.**

A1: What is the likely differential diagnosis?
- Endometriosis.
- Chronic PID.
- No associated pathology (primary dysmenorrhoea).

A2: What issues in the given history support the diagnosis?

The patient's age would be against the diagnosis of primary dysmenorrhoea, which usually occurs in teenage girls. The combination of painful intercourse (dyspareunia) and painful periods is typical of endometriosis, a condition that is more prevalent in nulliparous women of higher social class.

A3: What additional features in the history would you seek to support a particular diagnosis?

Pelvic pain caused by endometriosis is typically cyclical and at its worst at the time of menses, but can start a few days before. However, primary dysmenorrhoea usually eases within 1–2 days of the onset of menses. Previous infertility and a family history of the condition may support the possibility of endometriosis. Endometriosis may be associated with bowel or urinary symptoms.

A4: What clinical examination would you perform and why?

Speculum examination may reveal spots or (blue) nodules of endometriosis in the posterior fornix. Bimanual examination should be performed to assess uterine fixity and pelvic tenderness, which might suggest either PID or endometriosis. Nodularity in the uterosacral ligaments is typical of endometriosis, particularly on the left side. There may be an adnexal mass associated with endometrioma (ovarian cyst endometriosis).

A5: What investigations would be most helpful and why?

- **Investigations for gynaecological infections** ☑ Investigations should be performed for infection if the history and examination suggest PID (see Case 11.2).

- **USS** ☑ A pelvic USS should be performed, which, although not specific for endometriosis, would exclude an ovarian endometrioma.

- **Diagnostic laparoscopy** ☑ The definitive diagnosis of endometriosis is established by laparoscopy. However, no pathology is seen at laparoscopy in 50–60 per cent of patients with chronic pelvic pain.

- **MRI** ± Particularly if deep tissue endometriosis is suspected, i.e. in the rectovaginal space.

A6: What treatment options are appropriate?

SUPPORTIVE

- Explain the nature of the problem. Endometriosis is not a curable disease.
- Monitor the disease and its symptoms by means of ultrasound or magnetic resonance imaging.

MEDICAL

- The aim of medical treatment is to provide pain relief and induce amenorrhoea. Endometriosis (and its symptoms) often recurs after cessation of medical treatment.
- Non-steroidal anti-inflammatory drugs (NSAIDs) should be given for dysmenorrhoea.
- The combined oral contraceptive pill given *continuously* for at least 3 months, but preferably for 6 months. If this alleviates the symptoms, the diagnosis is very likely to be endometriosis. This treatment regimen could then be continued indefinitely (up to 38–40 years of age) or until pregnancy is desired.
- Progestogen (oral, injectable or intrauterine device).
- Danazol, limited use as side effects include acne, hirsutism, voice changes and weight gain.
- Gonadotrophin-releasing hormone analogues (side effects include menopausal symptoms, which are treatable with add-back hormone replacement therapy). Long-term treatment without add-back HRT is not recommended beyond 6 months due to the risk of drug-induced osteoporosis.

SURGICAL

- Specific treatment of symptomatic endometriosis depends on the severity of the condition and the patient's desire for fertility.
  - Mild endometriosis (few peritoneal spots at laparoscopy, no scarring): surgical ablation or excision, which has been shown to improve fertility chances, possibly followed by medical treatment for 3–6 months (if fertility is not desired);
  - Moderate endometriosis (peritoneal and ovarian spots at laparoscopy, minor scarring): surgical ablation or excision plus adhesiolysis, possibly followed by medical treatment for 6 months;
  - Severe endometriosis (peritoneal and ovarian spots at laparoscopy, severe scarring, tubal blockage): surgical excision of endometriosis (hysterectomy and bilateral salpingo-oophorectomy if appropriate); medical treatment for 6 months as for moderate endometriosis after conservative surgery.

⚕ OSCE counselling cases

OSCE COUNSELLING CASE 11.1 – **I am having a diagnostic laparoscopy. Should I be concerned?**

A1: What information will you need to provide when counselling her about the investigation?

- Laparoscopy is being performed to look for a cause for pelvic pain. It allows a telescopic examination of the gynaecological and abdominal organs. It is regarded as an intermediate operative procedure and is performed as a day case, although it does carry risks.
- The procedure is conducted as follows: once the patient is asleep under general anaesthetic, CO_2 is introduced into her abdomen by a small needle inserted in the navel. This enables a telescope to be inserted via a small incision in the navel. The surgeon then examines the pelvic area and reproductive organs to see if there is any obvious reason for the pelvic pain, such as endometriosis. If this is the case, this may be treated surgically at the same time. If there is no obvious cause for the pain, no further treatment is necessary. The surgery does not usually result in any noticeable discomfort, and the patient can be discharged home a few hours after laparoscopy. There are two or three small cuts on the abdomen and may not even require stitches. If stitches are required, they may be self-absorbing so that they may not need to be removed later. There should be minimal scarring from these incisions under normal circumstances.
- Although laparoscopy is a relatively safe procedure, like any other surgical procedure, it is not without risks and side effects. These include possible damage to organs (bowel, bladder, ureters and blood vessels) inside the abdomen. However, the likelihood of such complications is minimal.
- If complications do occur, they will have to be dealt with by an open operation (laparotomy). If this is the case, an inpatient stay of several days postoperatively may be required.
- There are also risks associated with the general anaesthesia.
- A written information leaflet about diagnostic laparoscopy should be given to the patient to reinforce verbal information.

OSCE COUNSELLING CASE 11.2 – **I have had a diagnostic laparoscopy. What happens next?**

A1: What information will you need to provide when counselling her before discharge from hospital?

- The laparoscopy shows a completely normal pelvis. This is the case in 50–60 per cent of women who undergo laparoscopy for chronic pelvic pain.
- It is reassuring in that there is no evidence of endometriosis, adhesions, PID or other gynaecological pathology.
- This does not exclude other causes of pelvic pain, e.g. irritable bowel syndrome. Information on improving dietary fibre and fluid intake should be given.
- In the absence of organic pathology, no specific gynaecological treatment is required. However, further investigation of other possible causes of pain might have to be performed.
- If the two or three cuts on the abdomen have been stitched, provide information about how they are to be managed. Also provide information about simple postoperative painkillers, and reassure the patient that scarring from these incisions will be minimal under normal circumstances.

- After discharge from hospital, if the postoperative pain does not show progressive improvement, the patient must contact the hospital.
- Advise the patient about follow-up arrangements. If the pelvic pain does not settle in response to simple measures, assessment in a combined pain clinic (where an assessment can be made by a psychologist or anaesthetist interested in chronic pain management) may be necessary.
- Provide the patient with a written information leaflet.

REVISION PANEL

- In STIs, all attempts to contact present and previous partners should be encouraged.
- Incomplete treatment of STIs should be avoided as there is a high chance of recurrence with long-term risks, such as infertility.
- Chronic pelvic pain accounts for 15 per cent of all new gynaecological referrals. It has an annual prevalence of 38/1000 compared to asthma (37/1000) and chronic backache (41/1000).
- Endometriosis can be mistaken for symptoms similar to irritable bowel syndrome and interstitial cystitis.

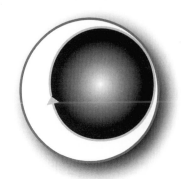

12 Infertility

Questions

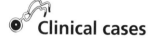

Clinical cases

For each of the case scenarios given, consider the following:

Q1: What is the likely differential diagnosis?
Q2: What issues in the given history support the diagnosis?
Q3: What additional features in the history would you seek to support a particular diagnosis?
Q4: What clinical examination would you perform and why?
Q5: What investigations would be most helpful and why?
Q6: What treatment options are appropriate?

CASE 12.1 – We are unable to have a pregnancy.

A young couple present with a history of inability to conceive despite unprotected intercourse for the past 2 years. The couple have had no previous conceptions. The gynaecological history is unremarkable. The female partner has had regular menstrual cycles without the oral contraceptive pill. The frequency of intercourse is two to three times per week. In addition, the couple have been timing intercourse according to an ovulation kit for the last 6 months. There is a history of mumps in childhood in the male partner.

CASE 12.2 – My periods are irregular and I cannot conceive.

A 28-year-old woman with a body mass index (BMI) of 30 presents with an inability to conceive despite unprotected intercourse for 18 months. Her periods are erratic, sometimes with 6 weeks between periods. She started taking the pill at the age of 18 years and stopped 18 months ago. Her periods were irregular before commencement of the pill. She has had no previous pregnancies, but her partner has fathered a child previously.

CASE 12.3 – I have been pregnant before, but I cannot conceive now.

A 32-year-old married nurse presents with an 18-month history of inability to conceive after removal of an intrauterine contraceptive device (IUCD). The IUCD had been in place for 3 years, was inserted after the birth of her second child, and was removed because of her wish to try for another child. Her periods are regular with mild dysmenorrhoea, and she is with the same partner who fathered her previous children.

• •

👫 OSCE counselling cases

OSCE COUNSELLING CASE 12.1 – **Is my coital timing correct?**

A 30-year-old woman has been trying for her first pregnancy for 10 months. She thought that pregnancy occurred around the time of menstruation, but has recently heard from a friend that this is not the case. She feels that she does not understand the best time for her to conceive. She has always had a regular 32-day cycle.

Q1: How would you counsel this patient about coital timing?

OSCE COUNSELLING CASE 12.2 – **Should my ovaries be stimulated to produce eggs?**

A 28-year-old woman attends for the results of her infertility investigations. These are summarized in Table 12.1.

Table 12.1

Test	Value obtained	Normal range
Luteal phase progesterones (ng/mL)	7, 12 and 9 on three separate occasions	>20
Prolactin (IU/mL)	300	150–500
LH (mIU/mL)	12	1.8–13.4
FSH (mIU/mL)	4	3.0–12.0
Rubella	Immune	–
Husband's semen	Normal	–

Q1: What is the potential reason for this patient's infertility and what first-line treatment are you going to recommend for rectifying this?

Key concepts

In order to work through the core clinical cases in this chapter, you will need to understand the following key concepts.

INFERTILITY (SUBFERTILITY)

Involuntary failure to conceive despite regular unprotected sexual intercourse for one or two years in the absence of known reproductive pathology (it is a symptom, not a diagnosis). After the first year a further 50 per cent of couples will fall pregnant in the subsequent year.
- Primary infertility: no previous pregnancy has been achieved.
- Secondary infertility: previous pregnancy (regardless of outcome) was achieved.

CAUSES OF INFERTILITY

- Male factor 25 per cent.
- Anovulation 25 per cent.
- Unexplained 25 per cent.
- Tubal blockage and other causes 25 per cent.

(Tubal blockage is more common when there is a high prevalence of pelvic infection.)

POLYCYSTIC OVARIAN SYNDROME

Polycystic ovarian syndrome (PCOS) is a condition in which the ovaries often produce more small follicles than normal, but the woman does not ovulate. It requires the presence of at least two of the following three criteria:
- Oligo- and/or anovulation.
- Clinical and/or biochemical hyperandrogenism (hirsutism, raised testosterone and dehydroepiandrosterone sulphate levels and reduced sex-hormone binding globulin [SHBG] levels).
- Polycystic ovaries on ultrasound with at least 12 subcapsular follicles measuring 2–9 mm in diameter and/or an ovarian volume in excess of $10 \, cm^3$. Other causes of polycystic ovaries should be excluded, such as congenital adrenal hyperplasia, androgen-secreting tumours, Cushing's syndrome.

Answers

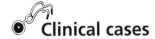
Clinical cases

CASE 12.1 – **We are unable to have a pregnancy.**

A1: What is the likely differential diagnosis?
- Primary infertility:
  - male factor;
  - fallopian tubal block;
  - anovulation;
  - unexplained infertility.

A2: What issues in the given history support the diagnosis?
Regular periods are usually a feature of an ovulatory menstrual cycle. The couple have been timing intercourse according to an ovulation kit, and it should be confirmed that intercourse is occurring before ovulation. It is unlikely that the cause of the problem is anovulation. Although none of the above factors can be confirmed or excluded from the given history alone, the history of mumps supports the possibility that a male factor is the cause.

A3: What additional features in the history would you seek to support a particular diagnosis?
A diagnosis of tubal block would be supported by a gynaecological history of vaginal discharge associated with pelvic pain. Pelvic pain may also be the result of endometriosis, which could be associated with tubal blockage due to an inflammatory process or adhesions. A male factor may also be associated with primary infertility, so information should be sought about general health, testicular descent, urethral discharge (e.g. associated with sexually transmitted infection (STI)) and occupational exposure (e.g. excess heat, smoking, alcohol and drugs).

A4: What clinical examination would you perform and why?
Obesity and hirsutism on general examination may indicate polycystic ovarian syndrome (PCOS). The breasts should be examined for galactorrhoea. Speculum examination might reveal discharge or infection. Bimanual examination should be performed to assess uterine fixity and pelvic tenderness, which might suggest either pelvic inflammatory disease (PID) or endometriosis. The male partner should also be examined, looking for signs of virilization, gynaecomastia, cryptorchidism, varicoceles, testicular size, and epididymal and prostatic tenderness.

A5: What investigations would be most helpful and why?
- **Rubella IgG** ✓ To confirm the female partner's immunity to rubella. If she is non-immune, rubella immunization (and appropriate contraception) is necessary.
- **Semen analysis** ✓ This should be performed on a fresh specimen after 3 days' abstinence. Any abnormality of semen should be confirmed on two specimens obtained at a 2–4-week interval, although

biologically, the optimal time for the second sample is at least 3 months after the initial sample because the cycle of spermatozoa formation takes about 3 months to complete. In the case of low sperm count and/or motility, additional investigations should include microbiological tests for infection, such as chlamydia infection, and an immunological test for anti-sperm antibodies. Sperm abnormalities should be investigated and managed by a specialist. Karyotype and hormonal assays (follicle-stimulating hormone (FSH), luteinizing hormone (LH) and testosterone) may be indicated as part of the investigation for oligo-/azoospermia.

● **Mid-luteal serum progesterone**　　✓　　This confirms ovulation.

● **Chlamydia infection**　　✓　　To rule out asymptomatic infection.

● **USS**　　±　　Depending on the history and examination of the female partner, a pelvic USS may be indicated to diagnose polycystic ovaries.

● **Laparoscopy and dye hydrotubation and/or hysterosalpingography**　　±　　If there is a possibility of pelvic adhesions caused by a history of infection, endometriosis or positive chlamydia infection, these tests may be performed to assess the severity of the condition and its amenability to treatment.

Female partner: Folic acid supplements to prevent neural tube defects.
Male partner: Specific treatment of male factor (oligo-/azoospermia) depends on the cause.

A6: What treatment options are appropriate?

MEDICAL
● Infection: treat according to cause, or empirically for chlamydia infection.
● Hypogonadotrophic hypogonadism: clomifene citrate or gonadotrophins.

SURGICAL
● Varicocele: high ligation of varicocele.
● Obstruction of vas: vasovasostomy.
● Donor insemination in case of azoospermia.
● Intrauterine insemination of prepared partner's sperm.
● Intracytoplasmic sperm injection (ICSI).
● *In vitro* fertilization and embryo transfer (IVF-ET).

CASE 12.2 – **My periods are irregular and I cannot conceive.**

A1: What is the likely differential diagnosis?
● Primary infertility:
  ● anovulation (polycystic ovaries, hyperprolactinaemia);
  ● unexplained infertility.

A2: What issues in the given history support the diagnosis?

A diagnosis of anovulation is supported by a history of menstrual irregularity that also pre-dates the use of the oral contraceptive pill.

A3: What additional features in the history would you seek to support a particular diagnosis?

A recent history of weight changes and hirsutism should be noted. A history of galactorrhoea would indicate hyperprolactinaemia. A past history of an STI and a family history of polycystic ovaries should be sought.

A4: What clinical examination would you perform and why?

Obesity and hirsutism on general examination may indicate PCOS. The breasts should be examined for galactorrhoea. A speculum and bimanual examination should be performed. The male partner should also be examined.

A5: What investigations would be most helpful and why?

• **Mid-luteal serum progesterone**	✓	Confirmation of anovulation is essential. As the menstrual cycle is irregular, the test should be taken weekly and the results interpreted in the light of the date of the next menstrual period.
• **LH, FSH and androgen levels**	✓	In PCOS, the LH:FSH ratio (measured on day 3 of the cycle) is >2. Raised testosterone and dehydroepiandrosterone sulphate levels and reduced sex hormone-binding globulin (SHBG) levels.
• **Serum prolactin**	✓	To test for hyperprolactinaemia. If confirmed, further tests (computed tomography or magnetic resonance imaging of the head for pituitary adenoma, and visual field assessment) for prolactinoma may be required.
• **TFT**	✗	Not required as a routine test. It is necessary only in hyperprolactinaemia, which may be associated with hypothyroidism.
• **Semen analysis**	✓	To rule out male factor.
• **Chlamydia infection**	✓	To rule out asymptomatic infection.
• **USS**	±	A pelvic USS to assess for polycystic ovaries.
• **Laparoscopy and dye hydrotubation and/or hysterosalpingography**	±	If there is a possibility of pelvic adhesions as a result of a history of infection, endometriosis or positive chlamydia infection, these tests may be performed to assess the severity of the condition and its amenability to treatment. These tests may also be indicated if infertility persists despite treatment.
• **Rubella IgG**	✓	To confirm the female partner's immunity to rubella. If she is non-immune, rubella immunization (and appropriate contraception) is necessary.

Female partner: Considering a diagnosis of anovulation:
- Folic acid supplements to reduce the risk of neural tube defects.
- Timing intercourse around ovulation (using an ovulation kit if necessary).
- Induce ovulation with clomifene citrate (see OSCE Counselling Case 12.2).

Specific treatment depends on the cause.

A6: What treatment options are appropriate?

MEDICAL

- Polycystic ovarian syndrome – induce ovulation. If clomifene is not successful, use clomifene and metformin (as this patient has a BMI of >25), gonadotrophins.
- Hyperprolactinaemia – bromocriptine.

SURGICAL

- Polycystic ovarian syndrome – ovarian drilling.
- *In vitro* fertilization and embryo transfer – a last resort treatment.

CASE 12.3 – I have been pregnant before, but I cannot conceive now.

A1: What is the likely differential diagnosis?

Secondary infertility:
- Tubal blockage.
- Unexplained infertility.

A2: What issues in the given history support the diagnosis?

The IUCD may have been associated with a clinical or subclinical infection that has led to damage of the fallopian tubes. Regular periods are usually a feature of ovulation, and previous pregnancies from the same partner indicate that male factor may not be involved. These factors would have to be investigated.

A3: What additional features in the history would you seek to support a particular diagnosis?

A diagnosis of tubal block resulting from pelvic infection will be supported by an obstetric history of deliveries associated with postpartum pyrexia and foul lochia, or by a gynaecological history of vaginal discharge associated with pelvic pain. Pelvic pain may also be the result of endometriosis, which could be associated with tubal blockage. Male factor may also be associated with secondary infertility, so information about the frequency and timing of intercourse should be sought.

A4: What clinical examination would you perform and why?

Speculum examination might demonstrate discharge or infection. Bimanual examination should be performed to assess uterine fixity and pelvic tenderness, which might suggest either PID or endometriosis. The male partner should also be examined for testicular size and varicocele (see Case 12.1).

A5: What investigations would be most helpful and why?

- **Laparoscopy and dye hydrotubation and/or hysterosalpingography**   ☑   To assess for tubal blockage, severity of the condition and its amenability to treatment.

- **Mid-luteal serum progesterone** [✓] Confirmation of ovulation is essential.

- **Semen analysis** [✓] To rule out male factor.

- **Chlamydia infection** [✓] To rule out pelvic infection.

- **USS** [±] A pelvic USS may be indicated on the basis of abnormal pelvic examination.

- **Rubella IgG** [✓] To confirm the female partner's immunity to rubella. If she is non-immune, rubella immunization (and appropriate contraception) is necessary.

Female partner: Folic acid supplements to prevent neural tube defects. Specific treatment depends on the cause.

A6: What treatment options are appropriate?

MEDICAL

- Pelvic infection: treat according to cause or empirically for chlamydia infection.
- Endometriosis: medical treatment for stage I–II disease is not indicated as it leads to delays in achieving a pregnancy.

SURGICAL

- Endometriosis: for mild endometriosis, ablation or excision at laparoscopy improves fertility and obviates the need for medical treatment.
- Tubal block: adhesiolysis, salpingostomy, and excision of blocked segment and re-anastomosis. Success rates are poor.
- Assisted conception (IVF-ET) has better success rates.

⛊⛊ OSCE counselling cases

OSCE COUNSELLING CASE 12.1 – **Is my coital timing correct?**

A1: How would you counsel this patient about coital timing?

- Conception occurs around the time of ovulation, not during menses.
- Ovulation occurs 14 days before the onset of menstruation. Therefore, in a 32-day cycle ovulation occurs on day 18 (32 minus 14).
- Sperm can survive for up to 7 days.
- Eggs survive for only 24 h.
- Intercourse should occur before ovulation, so that there are sperm ready to fertilize the egg.
- The 'fertile period', therefore, lasts for 7 days (i.e. days 12–19 counted from the first day of menstruation in a 32-day cycle). However, as ovulation can occur slightly early or slightly late in different cycles, it would be reasonable to regard the fertility period as occurring 1 week before and a few days after the expected time of ovulation.
- Abstinence is not beneficial. As long as intercourse occurs every 48–72 h during the fertile period, sperm will be in the vicinity of the egg at around the time of ovulation.
- The likelihood of pregnancy in any one cycle is 15–25 per cent (not 100 per cent) even in a perfectly normal (fertile) couple having intercourse at the right time.

OSCE COUNSELLING CASE 12.2 – **Should my ovaries be stimulated to produce eggs?**

A1: What is the potential reason for this patient's infertility and what first-line treatment are you going to recommend for rectifying this?

- The three luteal phase progesterones are low, indicating that anovulation is the most likely cause of infertility. The LH:FSH ratio is likely to indicate the diagnosis of polycystic ovaries but is now not considered the only diagnostic criteria. Additional features seen on USS and raised androgen levels are now important for PCOS (see Key concepts section).
- The first-line therapy for ovulation induction is clomifene citrate.
- The starting dose is 50 mg/day from day 2 to day 6 of the patient's menstrual cycle. A progesterone level in the luteal phase should be checked in order to evaluate the response to treatment. Intercourse should be timed, using a home ovulation kit if necessary.
- If there is no response to treatment, the dose of clomifene citrate can be increased by 50 mg in the subsequent cycle, going up to a maximum of 150 mg/day. Treatment should be for a maximum of 12 months. This regimen usually leads to ovulation, but pregnancy is achieved in only 50 per cent of cases. Pregnancy loss occurs in about 20 per cent of cases, so it cannot be guaranteed that the mother will have a baby even if pregnancy is achieved.
- The risks of clomifene treatment are multiple pregnancy (5 per cent risk and, therefore, ultrasound monitoring should be used) with associated poor pregnancy outcome and hyperstimulation of the ovaries (rare). There is an association with ovarian cancer and prolonged use is, therefore, inadvisable.
- If clomifene treatment is unsuccessful, ovulation may be induced with gonadotrophins, and assisted conception techniques may be required. Laparoscopic ovarian drilling is an alternative because it is as effective as gonadotrophin treatment and is not associated with an increased risk of multiple pregnancy. However, adoption, fostering and a child-free life are other alternatives.

REVISION PANEL

- In the general population (which includes people with fertility problems), it is estimated that 84 per cent of women would conceive within 1 year of regular unprotected sexual intercourse. This rises cumulatively to 92 per cent after 2 years and 93 per cent after 3 years.
- Coitus every 2–3 days is likely to maximize the overall chance of natural conception, as spermatozoa survive in the female reproductive tract for up to 7 days after insemination.
- Women (and men) who have a BMI of more than 29 are likely to take longer to conceive (or have reduced fertility).
- The use of basal body temperature charts to confirm ovulation does not reliably predict ovulation and is not recommended.
- Women who smoke are likely to have reduced their fertility (including passive smoking), which is likely to affect their chance of conceiving. Likewise there is an association between smoking and excessive alcohol intake (>4 units per day), which is detrimental to semen quality in men.

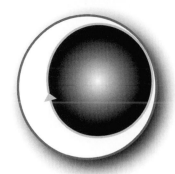

13 Fertility control

Questions

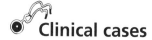

Clinical cases

For each of the case scenarios given, consider the following:

> **Q1**: What issues in the given history have implications for the request?
> **Q2**: What additional features in the history would you seek to support her request?
> **Q3**: What clinical examination would you perform and why?
> **Q4**: What investigations would be most helpful and why?
> **Q5**: What treatment options are appropriate?

CASE 13.1 – I had unprotected intercourse last night and wish for contraception.

A 32-year-old woman has unprotected intercourse during mid-cycle and comes to the family planning clinic seeking advice for contraception. She is also in need of reliable long-term contraception because she wishes to delay her family for at least 3 years. She smokes 10 cigarettes a day.

CASE 13.2 – My family is complete and I now wish to be sterilized.

A 27-year-old woman with three children requests sterilization. She has three sons aged 7, 5 and 3 years. She has been using the oral contraceptive pill since her last child was born. She has recently separated from her husband after a 10-year marriage and she feels that she does not want to have any more children. She does not currently have a sexual partner.

CASE 13.3 – I am pregnant and don't want to be.

A 22-year-old woman finds out that she is pregnant. She is not in a stable relationship and she requests termination of pregnancy. She was using condoms for contraception and she has not had any previous pregnancies.

CASE 13.4 – I have just had a baby and I now require contraception.

A 38-year-old woman had a normal delivery 14 days ago and is fully breast-feeding without supplementation. This is her second child and the two pregnancies were narrowly spaced. She previously became pregnant within 2 months of using the progesterone-only pill. She now wishes to have reliable contraception.

👥 OSCE counselling cases

OSCE COUNSELLING CASE 13.1 – How should I take 'morning-after' pills?

A 17-year-old university student presents on the morning after having had a condom 'accident'. She is extremely concerned about the possibility of pregnancy, which she feels would be a disaster at this stage in her life. Her last menstrual period was 15 days previously and she has a regular cycle. You decide to prescribe emergency hormonal contraception.

Q1: What instructions would you give her?

OSCE COUNSELLING CASE 13.2 – How should I take the pill?

A young single nulliparous girl is requesting the combined oral contraceptive (COC) pill. She has never used contraception before and has no contraindications for use.

Q1: Explain to her how to take the pill and give her any additional information about missed pills.

Answers

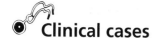

Clinical cases

CASE 13.1 – I had unprotected intercourse last night and wish for contraception.

A1: What issues in the given history have implications for the request?

Emergency contraception is not a substitute for a reliable long-acting reversible contraceptive (LARC) method.

A2: What additional features in the history would you seek to support her request?

It is important to establish the timing of intercourse because this will determine the type of postcoital contraception that would be suitable for the patient. Her sexual history, including the number of partners (and including casual relationships), should also be sought in order to determine her risk of sexually transmitted infections (STIs).

A3: What clinical examination would you perform and why?

If there is a risk of an STI, specific examination of the vagina and cervix will be necessary (see Case 12.2).

A4: What investigations would be most helpful and why?

If there is a risk of an STI, specific investigations such as high vaginal and cervical swabs will be needed (see Case 11.2). Otherwise, pelvic examination is not necessary.

A5: What treatment options are appropriate?

Emergency contraception:
- The 'morning-after pill' reduces the likelihood of conception at mid-cycle from 15–25 per cent to 1 per cent. It has to be taken within 72 h of the time of last unprotected intercourse. However, hormonal preparations are more effective if they are taken within 24 h, rather than 72 h.
- The 'Yuzpe regimen': two tablets of a combined oral contraceptive pill (equivalent to 100 μg ethinyloestradiol and 500 μg levonorgestrel) are taken, and the dose is repeated 12 h later. Prevents 57 per cent (95 per cent CI 39–71 per cent) of expected pregnancies. It is now not recommended to use this regimen.
- Progesterone-only pills: 0.75 mg levonorgestrel repeated 12 h later prescribed within 72 h of intercourse. This method prevents 85 per cent (95 per cent CI 74–93 per cent) of expected pregnancies. Nausea and vomiting are significantly less frequent with the levonorgestrel regimen compared to Yuzpe regimen.
- Levonelle One Step has now replaced the two tablet 12-h apart regimen (above) and contains 1.5 mg levonorgestrel given as a single dose within 72 h of intercourse.
- Newer methods are now available: EllaOne, 30 mg ulipristal acetate (synthetic progesterone receptor modulator) given within 5 days of intercourse, which has a primary mode of action of inhibiting or delaying ovulation.
- If the patient presents after 72 h, but within 5 days of intercourse, insertion of an intrauterine contraceptive device (IUCD) will usually prevent implantation.

CASE 13.2 – **My family is complete and I now wish to be sterilized.**

A1: What issues in the given history have implications for the request?

The peak age for sterilization requests is between 30 and 34 years. The patient's young age, all male children and recent separation from her husband are factors that could lead her to regret her decision in the future. It is possible that she may have made this decision in reaction to her separation. She might change her mind if she was to be reconciled with her husband or found a new partner.

A2: What additional features in the history would you seek to support her request?

Is the patient absolutely certain about her request? The history is targeted to determine the patient's fitness for anaesthesia, to make a choice of operative approach in the light of previous operations, and to explore the cervical smear history. The patient's last menstrual period date should be checked on the day of her admission to ensure that she is not pregnant before surgery.

A3: What clinical examination would you perform and why?

A cardiovascular and respiratory examination should be performed to assess fitness for anaesthesia. Examination of the abdomen should be made for surgical scars that may increase the risk of intra-abdominal adhesions and surgical complications.

A4: What investigations would be most helpful and why?

● **FBC**	±	Now not required in low-risk women for the assessment of fitness for anaesthesia.
● **Urinary pregnancy test**	✓	To exclude pregnancy at the time of admission to hospital before surgery.
● **Cervical smear**	✓	If not done during the last 3 years.

Table 13.1 Long-term contraception

	Advantages	Disadvantages	Mode of action	Failure rates per 100 women years (PEARL index[a])	Other comments
Combined oral contraceptive (COC) pill	Good cycle control, reduces menses flow, reduces dysmenorrhoea, and is well accepted. Risks of endometrial and ovarian cancer and endometriosis are reduced. There is also a reduction in morbidity of rheumatoid arthritis and thyroid disorders	Higher doses have a higher risk of venous thromboembolism, particularly if the woman is a smoker (see below). Also not suitable for those aged over 40 years, and for hypertensive and overweight women. Does not protect against STIs	Inhibits ovulation by suppressing LH and FSH release	0.16–0.27	Would be suitable for this patient (possibly with condoms to reduce her risk from STIs)
Progesterone-only pill (POP)	Safe to use in older women and following pregnancy in lactating women. There are no increased risks of thrombosis	Daily tablet, meticulous timing (±3 h) is extremely important for it to be effective. Does not protect against STIs	Cervical mucus becomes hostile to sperm and can inhibit ovulation in up to 40 per cent of women	2–3	Depot progestogens have similar mode of action to POP. Injection every 3 months means that compliance is excellent. Can result in initial troublesome irregular bleeding patterns, but causes prolonged amenorrhoea after long-term use
Intrauterine contraceptive device (IUCD)	Highly effective and once-only preparation, needing to be changed from every 3 years (copper) to 5 years (progestogen intrauterine system – Mirena). Latter reduces menstrual blood loss with up to 97 per cent of cases being amenorrhoeic within 12 months	Both types can result in pelvic infection and perforation	Prevents implantation and, therefore, considered by some to be an abortifacient	0.2–0.3	Mirena coil can cause irregular bleeding for up to 6–9 months

Condoms	Protects against all types of STIs. Essential for casual sexual encounters	Higher failure rate if not used properly	Barrier method of contraception	3.6
Cap/diaphragm	Woman has control over contraception, and the method is non-hormonal	Needs well-motivated individual to use it properly. Needs to be inserted before intercourse and removed at least 6 h later. Inconvenient to use and provides limited protection against STIs	Barrier method of contraception	Up to 20
Natural	Lactation has a major contraceptive role worldwide, as well as having major benefits for the neonate and infant (see OCSE Counselling Case 6.1)	Unreliable and offers no protection against STIs	'Rhythm' method avoids intercourse during the fertile period around ovulation, i.e. duration depending on maximum sperm (7 days) and ovum (24 h) survival (see OSCE Counselling Case 12.1). 'Withdrawal' involves removal of penis before ejaculation, but sperm can be released before orgasm	Up to 30

a If the PEARL index is 4, of 100 women using it for a year, 4 will be pregnant by the end of the year.
FSH, follicle-stimulating hormone; LH, luteinizing hormone; STI, sexually transmitted infection.

Table 13.2 Disadvantages of the combined oral contraceptive (COC) pill

	Incidence of thromboembolism per 100 000 women/year using COC pill
All women not using 'pill'	5
Pregnant women	60
Women using older 30 μg pill	15 (second-generation pill containing levonorgestrel)
Women using new 30 μg pill	25 (third-generation pill containing desogestrel or gestodene)
Women smoking and using pill	60

A5: What treatment options are appropriate?

CONSENT AND COUNSELLING

- It must be stressed that the sterilization operation is a permanent and irreversible procedure.
- In general, a 1:200 (0.5 per cent) failure risk is present. In the case of sterilization failure, it is more likely to be an ectopic pregnancy.
- There are newer hysteroscopic sterilization methods available (ESSURE and Adiana), which can be performed in the outpatient clinic setting using local anaesthesia.
- The traditional method is a general anaesthetic day-case procedure using a laparoscopic technique. It involves two small abdominal scars – subumbilical and suprapubic (or iliac fossa). There may be shoulder-tip pain resulting from referred pain from diaphragmatic irritation secondary to abdominal distension with carbon dioxide.
- Although the procedure is very safe, there are inherent risks associated with laparoscopic surgery – primarily visceral damage to bowel (1.6–1.8 in 1000 cases), bladder and blood vessels (1 in 1000 cases), which may warrant a midline laparotomy. Consent must, therefore, be obtained for a laparotomy in the event of complications.
- Check that the patient is certain of her request, despite knowing that sterilization will not stabilize an insecure marriage.
- Alternative long-term effective, but reversible, forms of contraception are available (e.g. IUCD).
- It is possible that the patient will experience heavier periods after stopping the oral contraceptive pill.
- If the couple had still been together, it would have been better to obtain consent from both partners and to advise them that the alternative is vasectomy, which is a quicker procedure, performed under local anaesthesia. However, failure rates are higher.
- Agreement to sterilization must never be a prior condition for agreement to undertake termination of pregnancy.
- Childbirth and abortion are both stressful times for the patient, and extra care and time must be given to allow her to reflect on the sterilization decision at these times.

THE PROCEDURE

Laparoscopic sterilization is a day-case procedure which should be carried out using the Filshie clip (2.7/1000 as it has the lowest failure rate.) Other methods have been used but are now not recommended: Falope ring (17.7/1000), unipolar (7.5/1000) and bipolar diathermy (24.8/1000). The patient should be advised to use the current form of contraception until the start of the next period after sterilization.

CASE 13.3 – I am pregnant and don't want to be.

A1: What issues in the given history have implications for the request?

A request for termination of an unplanned and unwanted pregnancy (therapeutic abortion) is a common request. This is usually a result of either poor motivation to use contraceptives or failure of contraception.

Reliable contraceptive advice and counselling would, therefore, be mandatory because abortion should never be used as a method of contraception.

A2: What additional features in the history would you seek to support her request?

It would be essential to obtain information about the date of the last normal menstrual period, the menstrual history and cycle regularity in order to establish a gestational age (see Case 1.1). A history of asthma would preclude the use of prostaglandins as a treatment option.

A3: What clinical examination would you perform and why?

If surgical termination of pregnancy is anticipated, the chest should be examined to assess fitness for anaesthesia. Abdominal examination would also be necessary in order to determine uterine size. A palpable uterus on abdominal examination would indicate a gestation of more than 12 weeks.

A4: What investigations would be most helpful and why?

● **FBC**	±	Now not required in low-risk women for the assessment of fitness for anaesthesia.
● **Blood group**	✓	To check the patient's rhesus status (if she is rhesus negative, prophylactic anti-D will be required).
● **USS**	✓	To determine the gestational age accurately.

A5: What treatment options are appropriate?

CONSENT AND COUNSELLING

- It should be made clear that there is a risk of infertility after an abortion, which could lead to considerable psychological trauma in the future. Psychological morbidity and regret can be considerable, and counselling should be offered as part of the termination service. There is evidence that this psychological morbidity is lower in women who choose medical methods of abortion.
- The complication rates are lower with medical methods, particularly the risk of sepsis (which can lead to future infertility). Perforation of the uterus and visceral damage can occur with surgical methods, but are rare and dependent on the surgeon's expertise.
- The risk of pregnancy is highest in the first 4 weeks after an abortion, and thus adequate contraceptive advice, such as the COC pill, depot progestogens or IUCD, is mandatory. This contraception should preferably be started before the patient is discharged.

The treatment options are as follows:

MEDICAL

- Up to 9 weeks' gestation – oral mifepristone (an anti-progesterone abortifacient) followed by vaginal prostaglandins administered 24–48 h later would result in complete abortion in 95 per cent of cases. The earlier the gestation, the higher the probability of complete abortion.
- A gestation of 6 weeks or less – surgical abortion would not be advisable because the pregnancy can be missed. However, before this method is considered, an ultrasound dating of the pregnancy is essential to ensure that the pregnancy is less than 9 completed weeks.

SURGICAL

Surgical evacuation of the uterus, normally with a suction curette, is the most common method of terminating pregnancy, and is usually performed as a day-case procedure under general anaesthesia.

Local anaesthesia procedures have now been developed. This procedure is safe up to 12 weeks' gestation. In nulliparous women, cervical 'ripening' agents (e.g. prostaglandins, mifepristone) are essential to soften the cervix before cervical dilatation in order to reduce the risk of trauma to the cervix and potential cervical incompetence in the future. The administration of prophylactic antibiotics at the time of termination of pregnancy reduces post-abortal pelvic infection.

CASE 13.4 – I have just had a baby and I now require contraception.

A1: What issues in the given history have implications for the request?

Breast-feeding (lactational amenorrhoea method) is the most common type of contraception used worldwide. It works by preventing ovulation and causing amenorrhoea. Fully breast-feeding without supplementation provides more than 98 per cent protection until one of three conditions occur: menses return, breast-feeding frequency is reduced or the baby reaches 6 months of age. This patient requires a more reliable form of contraception than full breast-feeding. The progesterone-only pill is safe to use in lactating women, but is effective only if it is taken religiously. It can cause irregularity of the cycle, which can result in non-compliance. This method failed after the patient's last pregnancy. Thus, another reliable form of contraception is necessary to reduce the risk of an unwanted pregnancy. It is possible that ovulation can occur before the menses and, therefore, it is essential to prescribe a more effective form of contraception almost immediately. The patient's age and the fact that she is breast-feeding are significant factors to consider when choosing an appropriate contraceptive. The COC pill is contraindicated in women who are breast-feeding and it suppresses lactation.

A2: What additional features in the history would you seek to support her request?

A history of smoking and obesity would increase the patient's risk of venous thromboembolism if she were to be prescribed the COC pill. Enquire whether the patient's family is complete because she might then be a candidate for sterilization.

A3: What clinical examination would you perform and why?

No specific examination is necessary. Pelvic examination is required only if there are gynaecological symptoms.

A4: What investigations would be most helpful and why?

No specific investigations are required.

A5: What treatment options are appropriate?

Encourage full breast-feeding because it has many benefits (see OSCE Counselling Case 6.1). However, the contraceptive benefit of breast-feeding will not be sufficient for this patient. Any of the methods described below will be suitable for her:

- Depot progestogens (Depo-Provera): this is a 3-month form of contraception and it is effective if compliance is going to be a problem. It is safe to prescribe for women who are breast-feeding. It can also be used to avoid pregnancy after postnatal rubella immunization. It can cause irregular bleeding and prolonged amenorrhoea.
- IUCD: this is highly effective, particularly in poorly compliant women. It is a LARC and it is suitable for older women. It can normally be placed after delivery of the placenta or 6 weeks postnatally. There is a higher probability of expulsion in the former case because the uterus contracts rapidly postnatally. There is also a risk of perforation (caused by a soft uterus) and infection in the immediate postpartum period.

- Sterilization: when performed after 3 months following delivery, this is known as 'interval laparoscopic sterilization'. If performed immediately postnatally, it would require a mini-laparotomy procedure because the uterus is still enlarged to between 14 and 16 weeks' size, which does not permit a laparoscopic approach. Filshie clip application and modified Pomeroy (cutting the fallopian tube) are equally effective (equal failure rates for both procedures [6/1000]). The latter method needs to be discussed with the couple during early pregnancy to ensure that they are completely happy about the permanent and irreversible nature of the procedure. However, the morbidity to the mother is considerably less at interval sterilization because it can be performed as a day-case procedure and also allows an adequate safe interval to assess whether the neonate is healthy before proceeding to a permanent form of contraception. Newer hysteroscopic methods, e.g. ESSURE, can be used in the interval period.

ii OSCE counselling cases

OSCE COUNSELLING CASE 13.1 – **How should I take 'morning-after' pills?**

A1: What instructions would you give her?

- There are two forms of emergency hormonal contraception:
    - the progestogen-only emergency contraceptive consists of 0.75 mg levonorgestrel repeated 12 h later. It is more effective and has fewer side effects (nausea and vomiting in 23 and 6 per cent, respectively) than the combined pill. It is the treatment of choice. A single dose of 1.5 mg levonorgestrel is now just as effective;
    - two tablets of a COC pill (equivalent to 100 μg ethinyloestradiol and 500 μg levonorgestrel) are taken, and the dose is repeated 12 h later. This treatment is now not recommended due to side effects and poorer efficacy.
- Nausea and vomiting are common problems (in up to 50 and 20 per cent of cases, respectively) with the COC pill. If the tablets are expelled in the vomitus, treatment may need to be repeated. An antiemetic could be prescribed.
- Advise the patient to use barrier methods until her next period.
- Warn her that her period may be early or late.
- Advise her that she needs to return for follow-up, whether or not she has a period or light bleed, to ensure that she is not pregnant and that she has effective contraception for the future (choosing one of the options from Table 13.1).

OSCE COUNSELLING CASE 13.2 – **How should I take the pill?**

A1: Explain to her how to take the pill and give her any additional information about missed pills.

- Explain how to take the pill:
    - start on day 1 of the menstrual cycle;
    - stop after 21 days;
    - have a 7-day break during which a withdrawal bleed should occur;
    - restart a new packet for 21 days;
    - give the patient a leaflet about pill taking.
- Mention the need for additional protection if the patient has vomiting or diarrhoea or takes antibiotics. This would mean using a condom for the duration of her illness or during the use of antibiotic treatment *plus* for an additional 7 days after.
- Indicate what to do if she misses one or more pills:
    - if she misses a pill during the first 14 days, she should take the most recently missed pill and use a condom for 7 days. Then continue as normal;
    - if she misses a pill during the last 7 days, she should take the most recently missed pill, use condoms for 7 days and start the next packet without the usual 7-day break;
    - give her a leaflet about missed pills.
- Mention the possible minor side effects (e.g. nausea, lighter 'periods').
- Mention the need for follow-up in 6 months, or earlier if she experiences any problems.
- Advise that the pill does not protect against STIs.

REVISION PANEL

- In the UK, contraception is widely available and unique in that it is provided entirely free of charge.
- LARC, e.g. copper IUCD or levonorgestrel IUS, is now recommended and is highly effective as is independent of user-related failure rates.
- Induced abortion is one of the most commonly performed gynaecological procedures in the UK.
- Around 200 000 terminations were performed in England and Wales in 2008.
- Over 98 per cent of terminations in the UK are undertaken because the pregnancy threatens the mental and physical health of the woman or her children.

Index

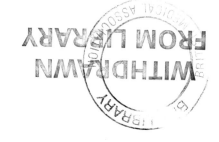